WELLNESS WARRIOR
FIGHTING FOR LIFE IN FABULOUS SHOES

LISA DOUTHIT

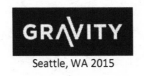

Seattle, WA 2015

Cover Design by Yosbe Design
Edited by Sandi Corbitt-Sears

PRINT ISBN 978-1-5137-0202-5
EPUB ISBN 978-1-5137-0244-5
Library of Congress Control Number: 2015951291

ACKNOWLEDGMENTS

Sometimes the English language can really let us down. There are so many words that beautifully depict what we want to convey.

"Thank you" is not one of them.

It seems trivial to plop these two awkward words into the hands of the people that have literally saved my life, but if that is the best our paltry dialect has to offer, I will give it a go.

First, thank you to my extensive medical team. From my neurologist Dr. Omidvar, Integrative Medicine Doctor Dr. Sadeghi, to my Internist Dr. Sandell and Stem Cell doctor Dr. Berman, I am forever grateful for your phenomenal care. I wish every doctor treated their patients with the skill and concern that you all do.

They say that if you put the prayer out there that you are looking for a guide, one will be provided. In my case that was absolutely true. I could not have traveled the road I did without the compassionate direction from those who paved the way for me. Thank you, Dr. Mikio Sankey, Mandaza, Issa, and my dear Mona Miller for showing me the way.

And finally, I am forever grateful for the love and unimaginable support from my family. I can't fathom what it was like for my then-young children when their mother was nothing more than a withered frame, feebly clinging to life. I'm truly sorry for putting you through that, but I am so proud of the strength and grace you pulled forward in that time, and the compassion you have towards others now. The three of you are amazing beings. I am honored to be your mother. And speaking of mothers, mine was a pillar of awesomeness then, now and always. Thank you for showing me how to "turn lemons into lemonade" and for always being right by my side my entire life. And to all the women in my life, I would not want to imagine what my world would be like without you. Especially my sisters. Individually we are strong, but together we are a force to be reckoned with. Thanks, Dad, for giving us the space to figure that out.

Last but not least, to my unbelievable husband Doug. "Thank you" is too lame for you. You were my eyes when I couldn't see, my ears when I didn't want to hear my fate, my strength when I was too weak to go on, and my voice when things got a little sketchy. You read my mind, felt my pain, and breathed new life in me when I wanted to let go. Thanks for believing in me and never wavering in your support and love. The feeling is very mutual.

*This book is dedicated to anyone who felt forsaken and abandoned in their journey with illness. May you always remember that you are **never** alone . . . **never** . . . **ever**.*

And to my kids Tanner, Riley, and Jordan, who one day may actually read this and think they should have listened to their mother.

And to my husband Doug, who took our vows, "For better and for worse, in sickness and in health" and embraced them with unyielding love and compassion. Thank you for being my warrior when I didn't have the strength.

Kintsukuroi *(n) To repair with gold: the art of repairing pottery with gold or silver lacquer and understanding that the piece is more beautiful for having been broken.*

FOREWORD

REALITY ISN'T REAL, at least relatively speaking. How can that be? We're all here in the world, and reality is the current state of how things are, right? Reality is just the way it is. Well, that depends on who you're talking to.

Reality isn't real because it's based on personal perception. Billions of people are experiencing life individually every day and coming to conclusions about the way life is that ultimately construct their idea of reality. Some people believe the state of the world is getting better while others say it's falling apart. Who's right? Which reality? It's from our personal experiences and often the influence of friends, family and the media that we create the absolutes (beliefs) that make up the filter of our perception. In fact if most of us look closely, we're likely to find that we've unconsciously adopted much of our idea of reality from the institutions and people around us. The point here is that because reality is relative to individual perception based on the life experience of each person, there are easily as many variations of reality as there are people on earth. It's impossible for a single set of conditions or conclusions to be labeled "the" reality because no two of us will have the exact same life experience.

If two people walk out of a movie theater and one person loved the film while the other hated it, what's the reality of that situation? Is the movie a good film or a bad one? The reality is, it's relative, based on the perceptive filters through which each person was viewing the movie. It's neither good nor bad; it simply is. Each person's reality of that experience will be determined through the perceptions they bring to it concerning the content, characters, storyline, and so on. Unfortunately, war is a constant occurrence in the world today and yet on either side of each war you will find a very different reality based upon the opposing perceptions of the events leading up to the conflict.

The good news is that because reality is relative, we can change our experience of it. How do we do that? We do it by consciously changing our perception of what's happening to or around us. The events simply are; they exist. We can, however, choose the kind of experience we will have by consciously perceiving the situation in a way that serves us. Death is a perfect example. When someone dies, one person may choose to perceive the experience as tragic and painful. Someone else may see it as a motivational reminder to live every day to the fullest as if it were their last, causing them to become more present in their life. This doesn't change the fact that the loved one passed away, but the shift of perception in the second person is what allowed him to create a different reality for himself that generated a positive internal response to the exact same event. William Shakespeare got it right when he said, "Things are neither good nor bad but thinking makes them so." We can't always control the events that happen in our lives, but we can take control of how we respond to them by becoming aware of how we choose to perceive them. In this way, we create a reality that serves us. If we think about it, our reality, and to a large degree our quality of life, is the collective result of how we choose to perceive what's happening to and around us moment to moment. That's all reality really is, a series of choices of perception from one moment to the next. This is why I tell all of my patients that how they relate to an issue *is the issue*, not their external problem.

Universal ideas of reality tend to coalesce when the majority of people use the same perception filters to understand something or a situation creating a collective perception. Again, so-called reality has nothing to do with the way something is, just the way most people have agreed to see it. This adopted reality has nothing to do with its inherent nature. We call a cloud a cloud because we've all agreed that's the word that should be used to name it, but we could have called it anything. A cloud really isn't a cloud; it just is. White is how we decided to describe how it appears, so that's how we perceive it. It doesn't mean that it really is. Collective perceptions were created for humans to have a way to communicate with each other. They're no reflection on the true nature of anything or how it really is. We could have easily described a cloud as green, and that would have become the reality of how a cloud appears to us. From this perspective, it's amazing to see how arbitrary so-called reality really is.

Some might argue that perceptions and judgments based on facts that can be proven and replicated create the fabric of universal reality. Light travels at 186,000 miles per second, and energy is equal to mass multiplied by the speed of light squared. These are incontrovertible scientific facts that can be replicated and yet, have no real impact on our personal daily reality. In fact, quantum physics would argue that light travels at a consistent speed simply because we perceive that it does and expect it to do so in every experiment. If we changed our perception to accommodate the idea that light could travel faster, it would thus create a new reality in which it did. In fact, some scientists are looking into the possibility that the speed limit of light does change, showing that even the scientific facts of reality are only limited by our perception of them.

In all of track and field history, it was thought impossible for a human to run a mile in under four minutes. No one in human history had ever achieved it, and the accepted reality was that the feat was physiologically impossible. Then in 1954, Roger Bannister ran a mile in 3:59.4. Once the perception of impossibility was shattered, a new reality was created. According to the *Sub 4-Minute Mile Re*gister, as of April 2014, 1,338 runners have also run a mile in under four minutes because their perception of what was possible changed.

Unscientific "facts" such as someone's account of a historical event or statistics are easily and often distorted for self-serving reasons leaving us with more misperceptions that skew our reality of the world around us and what's possible. It may be undeniable that some things exist, but the beauty of reality is that we get to decide what they mean for us.

Nowhere is perception more important than when it comes to our health. People have accidents, become sick or experience life-threatening illnesses. These situations happen, they just are, but it's the patient that gets to choose the context in which it's happening. I believe that mind, body and spirit are a single organism. An imbalance cannot appear in the body without a similar spiritual or emotional disturbance happening on a deeper level. Each plane of our existence informs and affects the others. With this in mind, I challenge my patients to change their perception of their illness. Instead of seeing it as an invader that needs to be fought with medication, treatment or surgery, I ask them to explore the idea that their intelligent body has given them a physical sign that a deeper emotional issue needs their attention and healing. Not only does this shift in perception alleviate much of the fear involved, it motivates patients to tend to their emotional exploration while I focus on the body. Perceiving illness as an ally instead of an enemy creates an entirely new reality for patients which places a difficult situation in a positive context and cultivates a more healing environment within their bodies. Getting sick isn't a conscious choice, but how we perceive the experience is. To make a perception change like this and enter into a deeper exploration of the heart and soul is to pass through the gateway to a higher level of consciousness and in doing so, eliminate much of the suffering associated with illness. Lisa Douthit made such a choice during her incredible health challenges and in her own words declared, "You may not be able to control the stream, but you can control the direction of your rudder."

Creating a new reality around how and why illness comes to us allows us to expand the idea of what healing is. We no longer dictate to the body what our healing has to look like. It can take many forms. In Lisa's case, she experienced a kind of healing that she hadn't expected at the outset of her journey and in ways that wouldn't have been possible without redefining her reality.

When someone receives a serious diagnosis and is contemplating their future, medically speaking and otherwise, they're often surround by well-intentioned but fear-driven people that urge them to be "realistic" about their expectations. Based on whose idea of reality? I tell all my patients that the last thing they need to be is realistic and sign on to the limitations others have collectively accepted. When someone says to be realistic, they're asking you to subscribe to and confirm their perception of reality for them. Because that version of reality is filtered through their layers of perception, it may or may not be true or even beneficial for you.

Even though life can be unpredictable, we still get to choose how we'll experience it through how we choose to perceive our personal reality. This unique ability allows us to understand one of the fundamental principles of life: you aren't in the world; your world is in you. Because of this eternal universal mystery, it's impossible to see the world exactly as it is because we've been created to see it as we are. To change your personal world and the world at large, you must change your perception of it first. Then you will find healing happening in ways you least expected. As French author Marcel Proust said, "The real voyage of discovery consists of not in seeking new landscapes but in having new eyes."

Dr. Habib Sadeghi
Agoura Hills, CA

STRIPPED

CHAPTER 1

It is not the strongest of the species that survives or the most intelligent, but the one most responsive to change.

Charles Darwin

IT FELT AS THOUGH medical problems permeated my entire life. As a kid, I would get strep throat and other typical childhood diseases, just more often than other children. In my teens, unexplainable rashes covered my body. They eventually went away, but when I was in my mid-twenties, they reappeared on my arms and stuck around for longer than I would have liked. After a few weeks and many failed home remedies, I went to the doctor, mostly due to vanity. After all, I figured, who would want to date a girl with red bumps all over her arms? For some reason, my doctor ordered a chest x-ray after studying the affected limbs. A week later, he called me back to his office.

I sat on the exam table, wringing my sweaty hands together in anticipation of his arrival. Doctor's offices have always made me nervous, and this one was no exception. When he walked into the room, he carefully avoided making eye contact. I thought that was rather suspicious, since he'd tried to ask me out during several of my previous appointments, which, I might add, was awkward during my annual gynecological exam. But I digress.

He mechanically placed a film on the x-ray screen. In a low, detached murmur, he said, "I want to show you your scan."

It was all he had to say.

It appeared fairly innocuous at first glance. After closer inspection, I asked why he'd used bad film, since it looked like there were shadows in my chest that resembled a halo.

"That's not a halo, my dear; it's a baseball-sized tumor sitting behind your heart."

And there it was, in all its disturbing and horrific glory. I'd gone in for some steroid cream to clear an unappealing rash and come out with a diagnosis of cancer.

Cancer.

Seriously? Who gets cancer at twenty-six? I'm no expert, but isn't cancer usually reserved for the golden years?

It was a surreal experience, to say the least. After my appointment, which had ended in silence and confusion on my part, I got in my car and drove for hours trying to understand how my world could be upended in thirty short minutes. Eventually, I ended up at my boyfriend's house. I sat on his front porch, completely conscious of the shock and emptiness I felt as I stared into space, absently holding a business card for a local oncologist.

A car pulled up to the house but stopped short of the garage. My boyfriend slowly came into focus as he made his way over to me with a questioning expression on his face. Judging by his concern, I must have appeared a little distraught . . . well, maybe a bit more than a little.

He sat next to me. "What's up?"

Looking intently at the tree at the end of the street, which seemed to be the most interesting thing imaginable at that moment, I vowed not to turn toward him for fear of breaking down.

"I'm debating."

He was confused. "About what?"

"Whether we should have Mexican or Italian for dinner tonight."

"Which did you decide on?"

"Mexican."

"We had that a few days ago."

"Do you want Italian?"

"I don't care."

"Obviously you do, or you wouldn't have commented on Mexican."

"No. Now I am dying for a fish taco."

I shook my head. "Let's do Italian."

"Okay. Italian it is. Anything else bothering you, honey?"

I vaguely remember telling him about the appointment with my doctor. I told him about the new path my life was about to take and that I had been "blessed" with cancer.

Blessed? Even I was not fully aware of the nonsense that slipped from my lips as I mouthed those ridiculous words. It was an odd thing to say, even for me. And I can say some pretty odd things.

I didn't realize it then, but looking back, I think the *I* who spoke wasn't necessarily the earthly *I* but the spiritual *I* we all have within us. There are many names for it: higher self, the soul, or the voice of God whispering in our ear. Whatever we call it, this inner voice was giving me a heads up that I was about to take a sharp left turn on the winding road of life. It was time to find my way down a different path or get off the highway.

My boyfriend's response to my "blessing" was, "When this is over, you wanna get married?"

I looked at him blankly. My brain was officially on overload. We had been dating only a couple of months, and, although the idea was lovely, I wasn't sure I was ready to tackle cancer and a marriage proposal on the same day.

Every girl fantasizes about the moment her man pops the big question. The circumstances surrounding his proposition just weren't part of my dream. Besides, I needed to keep my focus on the task at hand: ridding my body of whatever was eating me up inside.

Literally.

As the vision of a monster ravenously gorging itself on my innards crossed my mind, I started to wonder. Can this analogy apply on a deeper level, too? Was there something else eating me up, as well, that may have triggered a physical response?

No way. What was happening to the thoughts in my mind? Where were those ideas coming from? I'd always made fun of people who spoke in wild statements like that before. I believed in the scientific model and nothing else. Could it be possible there was more to understand out there? Was I willing to go *there* to see?

I supposed time would tell. For the moment, I would have to put those lofty concepts aside and settle for some eggplant parmesan and a cannoli.

Or maybe a burrito.

CHAPTER 2

SADLY, FROM THE MOMENT of my diagnosis, life started to feel like a bad movie I couldn't stop watching. After undergoing countless tests that revealed multiple issues, my fate was no longer in my hands but in the hands of strangers wearing white lab coats.

My thymus gland had gone rogue, expanding with disease and tripling its original size. Someone once told me that in the spiritual world the thymus gland governs compassion and inner peace. I had hoped to achieve at least one of those in my lifetime. Given my circumstances at the time, I wondered if those qualities would have been possible even with the gland intact.

Our new team of doctors explained that the only way to remove the tumor involved sawing my chest open and digging the diseased tissue out from around my heart. Unfortunately, when they opened me up, they also found lymph nodes in that area filled with non-Hodgkin's lymphoma, a completely unrelated cancer that is typically treated with chemotherapy and radiation. I later came to view surgery, chemo, and radiation as the trifecta from hell.

As the news spread to my friends and family, I spent much of my time listening to their well-meaning stories about other folks with similar illnesses who had *fully* recovered by eating nothing but kale, undergoing daily coffee enemas, and all sorts of other home remedies they swore by. Somehow, I knew my cure wasn't going to be that easy.

After months of tests and specialists, which led to three surgeries to remove various internal parts that my doctors deemed no longer useable, I counted down the remaining chemotherapy treatments and focused on a future after disease.

It happened so fast that it was all kind of a blur to me. Also, once we were on the cancer train, my new fiancé and I felt a sense of urgency to get married. It was like we were in some tragic romance novel where the tortured couple find each other only to be ripped apart forever by circumstances beyond their control. We were sure we could beat it, and together we would be stronger, so we expedited our marriage plans.

Every girl has an idea of what she wants for her wedding day. I had visualized myself walking down a long aisle in a beautiful white dress, with my guests looking on lovingly.

Our reality was a little different.

There was less than a week between my final surgery and the start of chemotherapy to tie the knot. We decided to elope, with a speakerphone by the pastor's side so my family could hear us say our vows from another coast. It wasn't the most romantic journey down the aisle, but it seemed to work for us given our time constraints.

Just like that, my dreams of a picturesque ceremony turned into a nightmare of hospitals, drugs, and radioactivity with a little break in the middle for a quickie honeymoon in Death Valley, California.

Looking back, I think we might have chosen a place with a more uplifting name. For those not familiar with this national park, it is situated at the lowest point of elevation in the United States. My new husband said he picked it because we had nowhere to go from there but up. I certainly hoped his prediction would prove accurate.

My calendar for the year went like this:

November 10 — Open chest surgery
November 20 — Implantation of internal port for chemo
December 24 — Wedding and short honeymoon
December 28 — First chemotherapy treatment
May 9 — Last chemo treatment
June to July — Radiation therapy
August 21 — Wedding reception
September 19 — Port removal
October 7 — Remission

In less than a year, my entire life had been turned inside out. In less than a year, I didn't recognize the person looking back at me from the mirror. At twenty-seven, my already-frail body had been pried open, dissected, burnt from the inside out, and filled with vile yet life-saving toxins.

Oh, and I was bald, twenty pounds lighter, and married. Not necessarily in that order but pretty close.

Was that the way a happy ending should look? I wondered. It wasn't quite what I'd imagined.

Finally healthy again, I felt I had been given a fresh start, so I forged ahead with my new husband and my new life. I just wasn't sure how or where I fit in any of it.

CHAPTER 3

CANCER PATIENTS experience a spectrum of emotions during their treatments, and I was definitely no exception. After the therapies end, the range of feelings can be even more diverse. You might start with elation and sink into depression in a matter of moments. There is a strong sense of determination during the cancer process to beat it, but when the battle is over, you can feel rather lost.

It's similar to graduating from college. You work for years to finally finish school, but after the big finale and celebration, you have a "Now what?" moment.

Now what? had become one of the top charters on my internal playlist.

Surviving cancer also brings forth conflicting feelings of cheating death and survivors' guilt, knowing that other comrades fighting alongside you have lost their battles.

Unfortunately, there is no information booklet on how to deal with all these contradictory feelings. At least I couldn't find one among the stacks of pamphlets I was given after my diagnosis. It also seemed odd to me that every brochure about coping with a horrible disease featured pictures of happy, healthy-looking people. No one I knew who was dealing with cancer seemed as ecstatic as the folks throwing parties on the covers.

Unfortunately, when cancer survivors eventually do reenter the human race, they become mindlessly distracted by routine jobs and the normal stream of living. We tend to forget about our new intention to change our lives for the better. It's akin to flipping the calendar to January 2. *What was that New Year's Resolution?*

I was no different, busily settling into my marriage and trying to forget the previous year ever happened. Sickness was replaced with mortgages and work responsibilities. My doctors told me children would not be an option because of chemotherapy, so I buried myself in the busyness of my daily routine.

I did, however, still spend plenty of time with specialists for regular checkups and multiple respiratory infections due to a very weak immune system. Many survivors tend to panic when they don't feel well anyway, so we run to all available medical personnel with any symptom that seems out of the norm.

For my thirtieth birthday, my husband decided to lighten the mood of our newly mundane existence by throwing me a surprise birthday party. Unfortunately, he was the one who was surprised. I felt sick with what I thought was the flu and couldn't attend. After a couple of weeks of feeling horrible, I quietly visited my oncologist to see if I was out of remission. After all, I was barely in year two of the five-year wait until I could be considered cancer free.

Even though I was becoming a classic hypochondriac, that time I really did sense a shift in my body that refused to go away. A feeling of dread came over me. My treatments rid me of the cancers but created many other issues. I was plagued with repeated cases of mono and pneumonia. Also, because of the chronic exhaustion I'd been feeling, I was convinced things were taking a dark turn.

Before making an appointment with my doctor, I'd already decided that the cancer had returned. I made a pact with myself that there was no way chemo would enter my world again. If the news was bad, I was done with the process and ready to check out of Hotel Planet Earth.

Did I mention that cancer patients can be rather melodramatic?

Or maybe that is more me, but my level of panic was certainly off the charts, which didn't help with my internal drama. I didn't want to concern anyone else until I knew for sure, so I kept the nonstop negative chatter and worry to myself for the moment.

A week later, I sat in the oncologist's office, waiting for The News. My palms were sweating, and I tried not to hyperventilate. I avoided eye contact with any of the nurses for fear of falling apart. They had always been so kind to me, and I knew if I talked to them, I was sure to cry. Fear can play horrible mind games, and my fear had become an ongoing theme once again.

Eventually, I heard the all-too-familiar shuffling of footsteps outside the door. Closing my eyes, I sent up a prayer to God, making a deal with Him. You know the "if/then" type? "Dear God, *if* you spare me the torture of cancer again, *then* I will go to church every Sunday or do whatever it is you want of me."

My doctor walked in just as I finished my somewhat manipulative conversation with the Man Upstairs. With my eyes still closed, I slowly turned toward him. After working up the courage to open them to see his face, my brain scrambled at what I saw. Instead of the gloom-and-doom expression I had come to expect, I was greeted with a huge smile. Instantly, I felt some relief, but the announcement he made confounded me even more.

"Congratulations, Lisa! You are going to have a baby!"

Huh? How?

Several doctors, including him, said it would be almost impossible to conceive after chemotherapy. I hadn't even considered the possibility of being pregnant. After all, sick people don't get good news in doctors' offices. What we typically hear are more prognoses and options involving protocols that make us feel like crap. I didn't have any idea how to react to positive information.

I was lost in my thoughts when I faintly heard someone say my name. The doctor was standing in front of me. "Lisa? Are you okay? Did you hear me? You are fine. You are just pregnant."

I am fine, just pregnant. I am fine, just pregnant. The phrase bounced through my brain like the words on the bottom of a karaoke video.

Pregnancy happens to normal people. Am I normal now?

* * *

When I was five years old, I sat outside my kindergarten classroom and listened as my mother talked with my teacher during the mid-year conferences.

The teacher had pulled out a series of finger paintings I had done. She said, "I am very concerned with your daughter's state of mind. I think she is very . . . confused."

"What seems to be the matter?" I could tell by her voice that my mother was both puzzled and concerned.

My teacher's tone took on an edge of annoyance. "We stress, especially to the girls in this glorious time of the Woman's Liberation Movement, that they can be doctors, lawyers, judges, even the President of the United States . . . pretty much whatever they choose."

There was a long pause in the conversation before my mother spoke again. "I'm afraid I don't understand."

"This is your daughter's painting of a girl in black on a broom. When I asked Lisa what she wanted to be, she said she aspired to become *Bewitched*. We are trying to teach her that she can be anything she wants, and she picked a witch on a television show. I think your daughter may have a screw loose."

I heard paper rustling, as if they were inspecting my artwork for clues as to why I would paint such an unusual thing.

I couldn't understand why everyone else wouldn't choose *Bewitched*, as well. After all, Samantha was beautiful, smart, and imaginative. She could fly and, with a crinkle of her nose, magic would happen. Who wouldn't want to do that?

Apparently, my teacher wouldn't. My paintings were never hung on the walls of our classroom for open house.

My poor mother argued that it was unfair to give a child the freedom to dream big only to judge her for her choices, but by then the damage had been done.

That was the first time I realized I was slightly outside the realm of normal and would probably continue to be that way.

* * *

My doctor was staring at me, bewildered.

"Lisa? Where are you? Are you listening to me?"

"I'm listening."

"Oh, and the rest of your labs are totally within range."

I had forgotten about the rest of my labs by then.

I paused to phrase my next question. "Am I normal pregnant or messed-up pregnant?"

Perplexed, he cocked his head to one side as his brows knitted together. "I'm not following."

"I am pregnant but not that long out of radiation and chemotherapy. Does that mean my baby will have three heads?"

It was an honest question. He searched for a few comforting words. He didn't find them.

"Well, I don't think it will have three heads, but I understand your concern. You haven't ovulated since before you started chemo, so we certainly weren't planning on this. It will be interesting. But you have always been an interesting case."

"Interesting?" I was not a big fan of *interesting* just then.

I wanted that perfect moment when I could shout to the world I was with child. My husband would be by my side commemorating each pregnancy milestone, and we would spend months in bliss as we picked out strollers and paint colors for the nursery. *Interesting* didn't fit into that picture.

"Yes, you may be high-risk, but you may be perfectly fine. Then again, you may miscarry. Who knows? All we can do is hope for the best and get you to a good OB/GYN. You never were within normal margins during your treatment; this is simply another beat on your own drum. Congratulations."

Congratulations. I am going to have a potentially messed-up baby . . . if I can carry it to term.

Glass half empty again or pure trepidation on many levels.

Will a pregnancy trigger my cancer again? Will I grow attached to the idea of motherhood and lose the baby anyway? Will I be responsible for someone's disfigurement because I had radiation? Will I be a good mom in the first place?

With a single word, I became paralyzed with fear. Again.

Cancer and *pregnancy*, two words that can bring you to your knees for very different reasons.

Do I fit in? Have I ever fit in? And what am I supposed to fit into? Why do we try so hard to conform when we should be attempting to break out? At least that is what I felt my soul wanted to do. My new life may not have had a storybook start, but don't most storybooks begin when the heroine meets tragedy and end after she gradually finds her way to glory? They say it isn't what knocks you down in life; it's how you get back up. I may never fit the perfect ideal of adulthood, but in retrospect, I'm not sure I ever wanted to. As Robert Frost once said, "I took the road less traveled by, and it has made all the difference."

CHAPTER 4

THAT EVENING, I BROKE the news of my pregnancy to my husband. He had the same bewildered look on his face that I must have had on mine. He, too, wasn't used to good news and was equally confused as to how to compute it in his brain.

Both of us spent much of that night staring blankly into space, but once the information sunk in, we decided to put all our fears on the back burner and try to think positively.

Did we have any other choice?

When constantly dealing with disease, you get used to life's struggles. You aren't sure how to handle the potential pleasures, especially when good news comes with footnotes. Fortunately, as the months rolled on and my belly grew, our anxiety gradually subsided. Once a few tests proved that a healthy, strong baby was growing inside me, and my own labs remained stable, we could finally move forward with a future centered on a family of our own to love. It was truly a once-in-a-lifetime miracle.

Or so we thought.

Our focus rapidly changed with our impending arrival. Doctor appointments shifted from oncology to obstetrics, and hospital stays were viewed with joy instead of dread. We bought a family-friendly house and sold our sports car for something more practical. A few months later, we greeted our tiny bundle of joy, a beautiful, perfectly formed baby boy.

Less than two years later, I gave birth to a baby girl. Eighteen months after that, we added another daughter to our quickly growing family. Oddly, my youngest was born on November 10, the same day as my open-chest surgery and tumor removal several years earlier. All of our babies were strong, healthy, and, best of all, completely normal.

After our last child was delivered, we realized the doctors had probably been wrong and chemo hadn't ended my ability to reproduce. We also understood that we should think about some protection if we didn't want to end up with a family the size of the Brady Bunch.

Taking my brood to my bi-annual oncology appointment, especially when I was pregnant, was great fun. Walking into the waiting room with my big belly leading the way and a stroller in tow reminded me of those post-apocalyptic movies where light deprived, tattered people come out of caves to gawk at the clean, shiny outdoor people. There was a sense of awe from the other patients that new life still existed in a world so filled with age, disease, and death.

Diapering, nursing, laundry, and cleaning filled my days after the children were born. It seemed important to prove to myself that I could do it all. I was determined to handle everything motherhood brought to me, even if it meant I no longer had time to eat, sleep, or properly take care of myself. Every minute of the day was filled with kids, cooking, and mopping up the mess. My husband was absent much of the time, trying to provide for our brood.

I was so busy surviving life that I forgot about my second chance to learn how to truly live it. Gone were the days of dreaming about fulfilling my potential. *Carefree* had been replaced with *confined*. Although I was grateful for my children and loved them dearly, I also felt slightly stuck in a life that had just happened.

I had no idea how my life's decisions were affecting my body and soul either. This journey was still not the one my spirit had intended.

I'd pushed the snooze button and fallen back to sleep after my first wake-up call. Something needed to change, but I didn't know what it was or how to get off the hamster wheel. Then fate took over and changed the trajectory of my course forever.

Again.

An age-old question asks, "If we knew then what we know now, would we do things differently?" Should I have taken a different path?

Was I even grateful for the chance to change? Probably not back then. But now, yes. Now that I know where my path has led me and what it means to live with intention, I am incredibly appreciative. The road I took has not been easy, but it has been interesting. My journey has taken me to places I couldn't have dreamed of before I got sick and pushed me further than I thought possible. It has also allowed me a chance to uncover the strength we all have deep within ourselves to rise above our circumstances and truly understand the deeper meaning of life.

CHAPTER 5

Smooth seas do not make for a skillful sailor
African Proverb

HAVE YOU EVER woken from a dream not sure if you were actually awake or still in the middle of it? I have spent years trying to understand where my reality starts and my dreams end. Many people have reoccurring themes or ideas in their dreams. I have had the exact same dream every evening for more than eight years.

Eight years. Who does that?

It always begins with footsteps. I watch my feet as I walk softly in the sand along the seashore. All is calm and peaceful around me. The sun is shining, and children are playing. I wonder for a moment where their parents could be. It's mostly babies wandering around and playing as if nothing else mattered in the world. To them, it probably doesn't.

I keep walking, lost in a trance of thoughts, simply following my own footsteps to see where they lead.

Feeling the shore beneath me, I notice the silence becoming more profound. It's eerie, like the calm before a storm. I look to see if the children have noticed. Unfazed, they tend to the castles and angels they created on the beach.

My thoughts ebb and flow with the waves until I feel the water slipping away from the coastline. The moment is all too familiar. Suddenly, a sense of dread overpowers my mind. Then I hear the familiar voice blowing softly in my ear, its subtle, ghostlike sound haunting me.

"Stand strong, Lisa."

I survey my terrain for the origin of the voice, but there is no one in sight. "Who are you? Why don't you ever show yourself?" I scream to the unknown source.

He continues, his words floating delicately in the breeze. "It's coming. You have to decide how to handle yourself. The darkness is about to envelop you. Make your choice."

"What darkness? What choice?" Questions that are never answered, just repeated by an unknown, unseen whisperer.

I sense imminent danger close by. Not completely understanding my situation, I search for the children who once shared the beach with me. They've vaporized, as if they were never there at all. Confused, my mind's eye hovers above the tide, detaching me from my body. I begin to panic. As I look toward the horizon, I see the peak. It is building, stronger and faster, heading straight for me. There isn't much time left, so I start to run up the beach, my footing unsteady. A dilapidated old house appears, and I stop for a moment to catch my breath and come up with a plan that will ensure my survival. I spot a rope lying on the ground. Running toward the house, I quickly tie one end around my waist and the other to the porch rail. I am terrified and hide beneath the shelter of the deck.

Finally, it hits. The enormous tidal wave that continually chases me, taunting me and threatening my very existence. All hope slowly escapes my being. I know I can't outrun the overwhelming flood, but can I possibly outwit it? Holding onto the rope, I gasp for air as the pressure from the water envelopes me. Desperate for survival, I try to barter with the ocean, hoping I can win it over somehow.

But there will be no bargaining today.

As I feel my essence slipping away, I wonder how I allowed this to happen. I also wonder what became of the babies who were playing so innocently. Was I meant to protect them? I ponder my own childlike innocence and think I should have better protected it, as well. My lungs burn from the saltwater, and I understand that it is finally time for me to cross over to the other side. It's also time to give up control of my own destiny. I take a final inhale, painfully filling my lungs with the fluid that has now consumed me.

Suddenly, I cross over, but I don't end up where I expected.

Instead of dying, I wake up to life.

It's always the same. The details change once in a while, but the main event remains consistent. I drown in a tsunami, waking up in a cold sweat just before I die.

I assume having the same dream for years must be a sign, a signal of something. But what?

I have heard that dreams come in different message forms. Some people describe them as a metaphor, others a vision, and still others communicate through sound or color. The way we receive information is as different as our thumbprints. I've spent countless hours trying to decode mine but to no avail. I've consulted books on dream theory and asked friends and family. I've even gone to a psychic to help decode it. Surely someone can figure out the symbolism before it is too late.

But the answers are always the same. The significance of the dream depends on its designer. I must unravel the mystery for myself. Frustrated, I feel like a child searching for a way home in a foreign land.

I eventually gave up my pursuit of the meaning and decided to collect the pieces of the puzzle, holding onto them instead of trying to put their fragments together. I may not understand what is going on in my psyche, but I hope that if I chronicle them regularly, they may make more sense later. Hindsight usually brings clarity if we pay attention to the details.

As soon as I'm awake, I try to record what I experienced and what I think may be the meaning. I pray that if I keep at it, an "aha" moment will eventually come, and it will make sense. After all these years, you would think I would have found clarity by now, but apparently I am not the sharpest tool in the shed. All I know is that the nightly vision is either a key or the foretelling of something really big.

And possibly really bad.

CHAPTER 6

Families are like fudge ... mostly sweet with a few nuts.
Author Unknown

WHEN I WAS TWO years old, my parents divorced. They were children themselves, barely out of college at the time of my birth, so to say my father hadn't had enough time to sow his wild oats would be an understatement.

My mother says the last straw in their marriage was when my babysitter's father came to our house, looking for him with a shotgun. You can probably guess why. She scooped me up in her arms, pointed to the hall closet where he was hiding, walked out the front door, and never looked back.

It takes a lot of guts to be a single mother, especially with no child support . . . or any other type of support, for that matter. She didn't complain; she just worked hard to make ends meet for our little family. We barely survived on her teacher's salary, but somehow she managed.

If there is such a thing as a genetic predisposition for courage, I definitely got mine from her. I sincerely hope that gene is passed down for generations to come.

A few years later, she married again but to a more grounded man who was just getting out of the military. He had aspirations of becoming an attorney, so we packed our things in California and moved to the East Coast, where he had applied to law school. Between his education, judge clerkships, and positions in various law firms, we moved around the country quite a bit for many years.

Attending eight different schools before college forced me to become self-reliant. Unfortunately, I missed the chance to develop lasting relationships. I was always the new kid on the block who watched lifelong friends share inside jokes. I tried to fit in at first, but I eventually retreated into my own mind.

I heard the adage "whatever doesn't kill you will make you stronger" when I was young, and it stuck with me. I remember thinking that I was the only person who could figure out my own problems. When I'd finally resolved an issue, I would say to myself (many times out loud) that it would make me stronger for when the really tough times hit. I don't know why I thought that at such a young age. All I do know is that I had plenty of opportunities to experience it.

Looking back, I think part of my make-it-work-no-matter-what mentality came from my mother, as well. Her favorite saying was "When life gives you lemons, make lemonade." Hearing her say it repeatedly made me crazy as a kid and even crazier as an adult, but it is forever embedded in my brain. Somewhere in my mind is a program that gets triggered whenever I run into "lemons." My ability to at least try making lemonade, no matter how impossible the odds may seem, has carried me through very dark days. It always gives me hope that somehow I can create something sweet from bitter circumstances and, hopefully, learn a little something in the process.

You have to exercise a muscle to make it strong. I think the strengthening of my spiritual and emotional muscles saved me in the long run. When things got tough, I knew I could handle whatever happened. Perhaps it wasn't my mother's voice alone. It may be that God's voice speaks through all our mothers, whispering in our ears that we will never get anything we cannot handle.

At least that was my prayer, because it seemed that He had very high expectations of my ability to handle what was about to be one of the worst experiences of my life.

CHAPTER 7

OUR LITTLE FAMILY of three grew substantially during my tween years, when my parents had twin girls, followed by my youngest sister, Katie, two years later. Living with four other females in the house and sharing one bathroom was challenging but a lot of fun. I was, however, grateful to be living on my own by the time they were teenagers. We were close growing up, even with the age difference. As adults, we are still best friends, trading clothes and stealing each other's shoes.

My sister Betsie, a nurse practitioner, became the family's go-to person whenever we had a medical question. She could diagnose anything from poison ivy to scurvy in a matter of minutes. Not that we ever had scurvy, but you get the idea.

Everyone should have a Nurse Betsie on speed dial; she was by far faster and more accurate than the Internet. I called her as soon as I returned from Mammoth.

My body was still not responding the way it should, and I was becoming concerned. No longer able to downplay the issues I was having, I promised my husband I would get checked out. But where do you go to have symptoms like "body acting weird" assessed? I figured Bets was as good a place to start as any.

When I called and told her the problems I had been experiencing, she sounded very professional. It meant she was in work mode and thinking of me as a case study rather than her sister with something possibly terribly wrong.

I could tell she was taking notes during our conversation. "So let me get this straight . . . first you started seeing double, and later you fell on the floor because your leg gave out?"

"Yes."

I prefer to keep to simple facts when we are doing the diagnosis part of our phone conversations. After we are done, we gossip or talk about our weekend activities.

"Anything else?"

"My speech was kind of funny, too."

"Define funny. Give me something I can work with."

"I sort of started to slur and stutter."

"When did this happen?"

"Wednesday."

"No, what time of day?"

"Oh. I think it was in the evening. Why?"

"I'm just making sure I record the information accurately."

"Any ideas?"

"I will call you back in a few minutes."

No gossip. All business. She didn't even mention the sale at Anthropologie. And it was a really great sale. That wasn't a good sign. Then again, it wasn't a bad one either. Neither of us had any money for clothes anyway.

For sure, she hadn't been very forthright with information.

Fifteen minutes later the phone rang. "I scheduled an appointment with an ocular neurologist at USC for tomorrow. It's at 2:00."

"A what? I don't even know what an ocular neurologist is. And USC is really far from home. "

None of it sounded like fun. All of it sounded alarming. *Tomorrow?*

It was happening a little too fast for me to digest.

"It's a four-month wait, normally. I called my friend at the doctor's office, and she put you on the schedule. You will be fine. Just make sure you are there a little early to start the paperwork. Call me after to let me know how it went. I gotta go back to work now; I have a patient waiting. Love you." And with that, she was gone.

I was very grateful for the nursing network; they really know how to make things happen. If nurses ran the government, I think we could eliminate debt and establish world peace in a matter of hours.

I was a little curious but mostly terrified as to what an ocular neurologist does. He sounded both important and expensive. And why would she set me up with one in the first place? What did she think was going on with me? Fear rushed through my body. I could feel my breathing start to constrict as if the weight of the world was sitting on my chest.

Am I really up for another medically induced fight for life again?
Is anyone?

Someone once told me it's the second thing that gets you. Confused by the statement, I asked for clarification. He was referring to an allergic reaction and explained that the first exposure doesn't bring on a negative response; it's the second. While the initial contact has no effect on the body, the follow-up can kill.

Cancer tends to follow a similar pattern. According to the American Cancer Society, secondary cancers make up the sixth most common malignancies. My second time around might not have been cancer, but it was just as malignant, spreading through my body and soul like a black shroud, sucking the life force from me. As difficult as my first war was, knowing nothing about the process had been a blessing. Knowledge can be a dangerous thing when looking down the barrel of another shotgun pointed straight at my head. The only thing I could do was pull the trigger and hope it wasn't loaded.

CHAPTER 8

The ultimate measure of a man is not where he stands in moments of comfort and convenience, but where he stands at times of challenge and controversy.
Rev. Dr. Martin Luther King, Jr.

SITTING IN TRAFFIC on our way to my ocular neurology appointment could not have been more stressful. The tension in the car was as thick as the smog and heat outside.

"Don't worry. I'm sure everything will be fine."

"Fine? Fine? You know how much I hate that 'F' word! Didn't we promise not to use that ridiculous word anymore? And you don't know everything will be *fine*!"

"I do know everything will be fine, because it always ends up being fine. And what will worrying accomplish, anyway? All we have to do is see what the doctor says and go from there, right? Relax."

"Relax? Don't tell me to relax! How could I possibly relax when we are driving over two hours away to a medical center for God knows what?"

"Look, whatever happens, I'm sure it will be fine."

"Stop using that word! I hate that stupid word! Like I said, you don't know that!"

"I don't want to fight with you right before we go in. I know it is nerve racking, but we have gone through this many times before. Whatever we find out, I'm sure we can manage this, too."

As I sat in the passenger seat of our car, I wondered why I was the one trying to calm my husband and convince him that all was well. Shouldn't I be the one who was flipping out? After all, I would have to go through all the medical procedures, and I knew firsthand how much they suck.

Despite my efforts to relieve his anxiety, he continued. "What if this is really bad? What are we going to do?"

Trying not to state the obvious, I responded curtly. "I don't know. I guess we will have to figure it out . . . if and when that happens." Our conversation was wearing on me. I was just as nervous, but we process things differently. He likes to verbally vomit all over everyone, while I like to hold it all in until I implode.

Neither is a great idea.

Wouldn't it be great if we learned in school how to process life? I imagine the divorce rate would drop significantly, along with number of folks in mental institutions, because we would be able to effectively communicate our thoughts and feelings.

The nurse at the physician's office greeted me with a warm smile and a stack of papers to fill out. Once I'd finished, she showed us to an exam room. Sitting in a special ophthalmology chair that looked a little medieval, I couldn't help wondering if this was all just a bad dream. Would I be waking up soon, or had my life really become this complicated, literally overnight?

One day I was packing lunches and doing laundry like most moms in America, and the next I was in another cold doctor's office, waiting for potentially devastating news from a specialist I didn't know existed just two days before.

How had that happened?

Suddenly the door burst open, and a crowd of people in white lab coats filed in.

"Hi, there! I'm Dr. Curious, and these are my interns and a Fellow, here to see what we can do for you today."

Dr. Curious and a Fellow? How seriously could I take a man who sounded more like an old vaudeville act than an important specialist?

I smiled and tried to make light conversation. Unfortunately, when I am nervous, things don't sound the same out loud as they do in my head.

"I bet you got teased a little in med school with that name." As I listened to the words coming out of my mouth, I thought I should employ a few more filters before I tried speaking again. From the look on his face, it was probably too late for that.

Am I the only person who blurts out inappropriate comments when uncomfortable? Possibly. At least I was in that office.

Ignoring my statement (thankfully), he continued. "I see you have had some trouble with your eyes lately. And muscle weakness?"

"Yes. It started a few days ago and seems to be getting worse."

"Did this happen suddenly, or was it a slow progression?"

"I woke up feeling fine, and it was like my body just disconnected."

He looked confused. "Disconnected from what?"

"Disconnected from me. In my mind, I'm telling my body what to do, but it just isn't listening. I would go to move or pick something up, and I couldn't. It comes and goes, but it is worse at night. I've been having trouble eating, too. When I swallow, nothing seems to go down my throat, and I end up choking. But I'm getting off point, because that doesn't have anything to do with my eyes. I've been seeing double lately."

He sat back in his chair as the interns wrote notes wildly. "I think your other symptoms may have more to do with your eyes than you think. I want to run a test on you where we inject a drop of medicine in a vein and see if your vision gets better."

"If that is all it takes, let's do it!" I was very excited about the quick fix. It looked like my sister had sent me to the right place.

He nodded, and I watched as the white-coated brigade marched out of my room and into the hall. I heard them consulting each other and directing someone to get the needed equipment for the test. A few minutes later, they all tumbled back in.

"Okay, Lisa. I am going to inject a drop of this medicine, it's called Tensilon, into your body. If it works like I think it will, your vision will correct itself in just a few seconds."

"Great! Let's do it." Looking around the room, I realized even more white coats than before were looking back at me. Suddenly, I felt a little stage fright. "Can you all talk amongst yourselves while we do this? You are making me nervous."

It wasn't nerves I was dealing with so much as the terror of having to deal with it all in a public forum. It felt as if they were waiting for the results of their experiment with a lab rat. And I was the rat.

They looked at my face as if they were seeing it for the first time. They were definitely much more interested in the procedure than in me and didn't move.

I just closed my eyes instead. "Go!"

He inserted the needle and administered the drug. "You have to open your eyes, or we won't know if the double vision is gone."

"Right. Sorry."

Ignoring the many bodies in the room, I looked directly at my husband. He was sitting in a chair across from me and smiling. Suddenly, his face went from two images to a single focus. Never had it looked so beautiful. "I'm seeing just one of everything! I'm cured! I can't believe it!"

Tears welled in my eyes. I quickly wiped them away so as not to blur my perfect vision. I basked in the moment while the white coats conferred with each other. Dr. Curious was telling them something in doctor talk.

That's when my vision doubled again.

"Hey, what happened? My vision is messed up again. Can you give me more of that stuff?"

He looked at me, confused. "No. That was just a test to see if you had what I thought you had. It confirmed it, though, so now we know."

"We know what?"

"We know you have myasthenia gravis. It is an autoimmune disease.

"Like AIDS?" That was the only autoimmune disease I knew. I was hoping it wasn't like AIDS.

"No. There are many different types of autoimmune diseases, and they are not all like AIDS. This particular one translates from Greek as grave muscle weakness."

"What exactly does that mean to me?"

He nodded towards the door, and the white coats systematically filed out of the room again. I wondered if they practiced marching in sync.

As soon as the door closed behind them, he moved his chair closer to mine. His voice was filled with compassion as he started explaining the terrible disease that now inhabited my body.

"Although myasthenia gravis, or MG, has been around a while, we don't really know much about how people get it. The hallmark of this particular autoimmune disease is muscle weakness that increases during periods of activity or stress and improves after periods of rest. Certain muscles, such as those that control eye and eyelid movement, facial expression, chewing, talking, and swallowing, are often but not always involved in the disorder. The muscles that control breathing and neck and limb movements may also be affected."

"What happens when breathing is involved?"

"I wouldn't worry about that if it isn't an issue now."

He had no idea who he was dealing with. I was the queen of worry.

A wave of panic swept through me. "Oh, my God, I have three children! Could I pass this on to them?" No parent ever wants to think her child will inherit something horrible.

He put his hand over mine as if to reassure me. "Myasthenia gravis is not directly inherited nor is it contagious. You didn't get it from anyone nor can you give it to your family. You didn't do anything to contract MG. You just have to learn how to live with it now."

My husband jumped in. "Surely there is some type of medication to get rid of it, right?"

The sound of his voice broke my trance. I'd been gazing into the doctor's eyes, desperately looking for something I couldn't find in them: hope.

He turned to my husband and said, "There is some medication we can try, but it is a little tricky, given her health history. You see, the typical protocol involves steroids and immunosuppressants, but those are two things one typically stays away from with a history of cancer. I am going to give you a referral to a specialist in neurology who works with other myasthenia patients, and he can better answer your questions. I know it is a lot to process, but with the proper medications, you may be able to lead a somewhat normal life."

A somewhat normal life. What is a somewhat normal life? On one hand, having an official diagnosis was a little comforting, considering my other doctor tried to send me for a psych evaluation after I explained my symptoms.

At least I wasn't crazy.

On the other hand, I wasn't very excited about the whole autoimmune concept either. My poor husband's face was ashen. When he took his vow to stick with me in sickness and in health, he should have put in a clause that specified how many illnesses he had to put up with.

Too late now, pal.

After handing us a pad of prescriptions and some eye drops, the doctor left us alone in the room. Fighting back tears, all I could say was, "I'm sorry."

He looked puzzled. "For what?"

"For getting sick again. You have been there for me through lymphoma, thyroid cancer, and thymus cancer . . . and now this? It feels like we have spent more than half our married life sitting in doctors' offices. You must be tired of this by now."

"No more tired than you must be. Don't worry; everything will be . . . fine." I looked up at him, and we both burst into laughter. I'm not sure why, but the "F" word seemed to come in handy at that point.

"I just can't believe how fast this came on. One day, I'm riding bikes with the kids, and the next day, we are sitting here."

Tears filled my eyes again as my voice turned to a whisper. "Do you think God is punishing me for something?"

He looked at me as tears streamed down his face, too. "I don't believe God punishes people. I do think this type of stuff can make or break you, though."

"What do you mean?"

"Lots of people just give up when faced with half the stuff you have been through. Marriages fall apart, too. We get to decide how we are going to handle this. Are we going to roll over and play dead, or are we going to play ball?"

He was always the sports enthusiast. "Play ball? What are you talking about? Do I have a choice?"

He smiled. "You always have a choice. You can become a victim to all the medical stuff you have had to endure, or you can become wise and strong from it. There is always a choice in everything we do, even if it is just how we are going to respond to it."

I thought for a minute about how ironic that statement was. "How does one become *strong* when dealing with a disease that literally translates from Greek to *grave weakness*? Isn't that an oxymoron?"

He laughed. "Are you kidding? We had to cancel our big wedding and elope so you could have open chest surgery, and we came home from our honeymoon early so you could start chemotherapy. You had three beautiful children after being told you would be sterile and made it through a couple other cancers, not counting all the skin stuff after that. You are like the damn Energizer Bunny. You just keep going and going. Good Lord, you have bounced back from chemo and radiation when you were so weak you couldn't sit up only to run marathons a couple of years later. Do you seriously think a little thing like this will keep you down for long? I think we will be—"

"You aren't going to say *fine* are you?"

Smiling, he said, "No. I was going to say stronger than ever. In ourselves and our marriage. Maybe I need to learn a thing or two, as well. Who knows, this may end up being the biggest growth experience either of us have ever encountered. Just know that, no matter what, we are in this together."

I started to cry again. I had spent a lot of time crying over the previous few days. He was right. As hard and impossible as it felt at that moment, we had already done many things that seemed hard and impossible, and we always made it through to the other side. And it had always made us stronger.

As I looked at my husband in the chair across from me, I thought about a time long ago.

*   *   *

It was my first week at my new job in sales. Like many young adults fresh out of college, I had just enough knowledge to think I could do anything but no real skill to back it up. Walking into my first real appointment felt like I was crossing the threshold of not just a new career but of becoming a grownup.

Sales presentation firmly in hand, I was ushered into the office of the president of the company. He was on the phone, but he pointed to the seat in front of his desk. I sat and waited.

And waited.

I tried not to seem impatient, but my nerves started to get the better of me. I had practiced my speech repeatedly the night before and was more than ready to present it to him. After he finished joking with whoever was on the call, he finally hung up and turned to me.

"Lunch?"

I wasn't prepared for that question. "Excuse me?"

He never broke eye contact. "Do you eat?"

I could answer that one. "Yes."

"Okay. Then can we do this over lunch? I haven't eaten today, and I have meetings all afternoon."

That was not in my sales manual, but I did have an expense account. "Uh, sure. I am new to the area, though, and don't know what's around here." I probably didn't have to point out my newness. I think he'd figured that one out by himself.

"I know a place. It's fast, and I haven't gotten sick from the food yet. You will have about twenty minutes to get this done there. I'll drive."

His charm underwhelmed me, but I was confident it was somewhere under all that ego. As we walked into the restaurant at the end of a boat dock, I wasn't sure what was worse, the smell of rotting fish outside or the pictures of nudes painted on velvet inside. The waitress wore a flouncy, semi-transparent nightie, as it was lunch-and-lingerie day.

Who knew that was even a thing?

After she took our menus, he looked at me. "Go."

"Where?"

He was getting annoyed. "No. Your proposal. Go."

Finally, it was time to wow him. Unfortunately, that didn't happen. As I pulled out my binder, the clasp opened and the pages fell out of the book. Reaching under the table to gather them, I tried not to touch anything on the floor. As I came back up, I hit my head on the table, knocking over a water glass.

My face turned red. "Oh. I am so sorry."

He looked for our server. "Can we just get our food to go, please? I need to get back to the office."

Nothing so far even remotely resembled the presentation I had practiced in the mirror.

We drove back to his office in silence. As we pulled into the parking lot, he looked at me and said, "Give it to me."

"Excuse me?" I wasn't sure where the conversation was going.

"I'm not interested in the proposal, just the numbers. If they make sense, we have a deal."

I wasn't prepared for that either. I wondered if I should rethink the whole sales position. My mother always wanted me to be a vet anyway. I handed him my cost sheet and watched him examine it as we sat in his car.

He quickly handed it back. "Okay."

"Okay, you like the cost analysis?"

Grabbing the pen out of my hand, he started marking up my papers. "Can you change this and move that over there? Also, I need to take delivery right away. You can make that happen, right?"

I didn't blink. "Of course I can." I had no idea if I could or not or what he was really talking about in the first place, but there was no way I was going to let him know that.

That was my first ever sales deal.

It was also my first meeting with my husband.

* * *

As I focused again on the cramped exam room, I watched as an older version of the man I'd sat across from in that car so many years ago tenderly gathered my things. Over the years, I had seen him change from angry and insensitive to understanding and compassionate. I often wondered how much my illnesses played a role in the change.

Many of us with health issues see ourselves as a burden to loved ones. Is it possible that there are some positive changes that can occur, as well?

I have certainly learned to love and appreciate those around me more than ever. Maybe he had, too. Could that have happened had I not gotten sick? Wherever MG was taking us, I was confident we would be in it together.

Well, pretty confident, anyway.

Hopefully.

CHAPTER 9

WE ALL HAVE OUR UNIQUE methods for coping with devastating information. Some of us are able to process through the experience right away and grow from it. Others retreat into denial, finding ways to avoid the situation.

Personally, I like to hide in my closet. It has a very comfortable floor and a little window that allows me to hear the birds on a nearby tree. It is also the quietest place in our house.

As I sat there contemplating another life-threatening illness, I seriously considered my options. I hated the term *options*; it's code for choosing between a bad or worse scenario. Options are never easy or uncomplicated.

All I could see in my mind was a ticker tape that read "autoimmune, smautoimmune, autoimmune, smautoimmune."

I never said it made much sense in there.

The "nice" thing about when I had cancer was that there was a beginning, a middle, and an end. Autoimmune diseases are not only life threatening but lifelong. Did I really want to take a trunk full of medication every day to feel a little better than lousy for the rest of my life? And what about the expense? Sometimes it seems we are all one illness away from bankruptcy, even with good insurance.

And we didn't have good insurance.

Then I wondered what kind of emotional trauma my family would have to endure with another ailment. How much is an incapacitated mother worth anyway? It wouldn't be fair if my children had to become my caregivers.

I could feel the bile welling up in my throat as tears streamed down my face. Was I even up for the challenge? I didn't think so.

Slowly, the life was draining from my body. I wasn't sure I even cared; I simply knew I was tired.

Really tired. To-the-bone tired.

That was when I heard a knock at the door.

"Mom? Are you busy?"

Was I busy? I was lying in fetal position on the floor of my closet. Yes, I was a little busy.

"Do you need me, honey?" I really hoped not. I wanted to spend a little more time feeling sorry for myself before I started dinner.

"I need some help with my homework."

Seriously? I was contemplating my very existence, and my daughter wanted me to proofread?

"Sure, Riley Pie. Come on in."

Or don't ... and let me continue to freak out in peace.

She flipped on the light and perched next to me, pretending not to notice my mascara-streaked cheeks and puffy eyes.

"I have to turn in this paper for English class tomorrow. Can you sign off on it for me?"

I tried to wipe off the clown-like makeup that had run down my face. "Sign off? What needs to be signed off?"

She looked annoyed. "I told you about this last week, Mom. I had to write a poem for school. The teacher wanted us to read it to our parents and have them sign off on it. Remember?"

Remember? Of course I didn't remember. I was too busy having a total meltdown to remember to sign an English assignment requested a week ago, along with the hundreds of other important details I managed before my life went completely to hell. Couldn't a girl flip out in the privacy of her own closet once in a while without having to finish the laundry or spell check?

Honestly! Did I have to do everything around there?

I took a deep breath and counted to ten. She was waiting for an answer, so I only got to five.

"Of course, I remember your poem. I know how hard you have been working on it. I would love for you to read it to me. If it is okay with you, I will sit back against my winter sweaters and close my eyes. The dust in here must be making them water."

Or maybe it was the fact that I had to look death in the eye again.

She sat next to me. "Ready? It's called 'What If,' by me."

What if?
What if everyone was perfect?
There would be no individuality.
What if no one had attitude?
There would be no personality.
What if no one had principles?
There would be no morality.

What if we all were the same?
Then no stories could be told,
Because all stories would already be old.
What if no one had their own kind of fun?
We wouldn't push on doors that said pull.
Everyone's life would be so dull.
What if no one experienced love?
Then it would be a feeling people could only dream of.
What if no one experienced death?
Then no one would have to take their last breath.

What if everyone was perfect?
There would be no individuality.
What if no one had attitude?
There would be no personality.
What if no one had principles?
There would be no morality.

I looked at her beautiful face, full of light. "That is beautiful, punkin. What gave you the idea to write it?"

She smiled. "You did, Mom. You are always telling us to run our own race and not be afraid of who we are, even if we are different from everyone else. It made me think about how boring it would be if we all were the same. Even when we are dealing with the same stuff, we handle it differently, and that shouldn't be something we are afraid or ashamed of."

I wondered if that included hiding in the back of a closet and crying because it felt like I was the only person in the world with serious issues.

Raising kids is a funny thing. You may think you are protecting them from the world's tough spots while trying to show them what life has to offer. But, in reality, I'm pretty sure it is them helping us navigate through the dark times.

At least that is how it seems to happen in my house. Just when I think I am at the end of my rope, they come in and throw me a lifeline.

I decided that giving up wasn't an option when there are people you love more than anything hanging around.

Looking into her eyes, I saw that there is always room for hope. No matter how dark things look in the moment, morning always comes in one form or another. I needed to release the inner victim that had taken over my mind and get it together, no matter how hard and overwhelming it felt. Besides, my life didn't belong to me alone. It was part of a much bigger picture.

CHAPTER 10

A man can be destroyed but not defeated.
Ernest Hemingway

IT WAS 5:30 IN THE MORNING and time for my daily jog. I love my runs, but part of me hates them, too. It's rough when you are tucked into your nice, warm bed only to be rudely awakened by an alarm clock telling you to put on some tennis shoes and hit the road.

Mile . . . what was it? Six? Seven? It didn't matter. Something about running along the beach makes me feel so peaceful, as if I could fly with the seagulls that flock around me. I rise before the kids so I don't have to worry about anyone else's agenda or what I should be doing. It's *me* time.

What is that beeping noise?

Probably nothing.

I'd recently read a book about Zen running and how people use it to learn concentration and contemplation. I liked the idea. The concentration aspect promised to be a good way to calm the chatter in my brain. Lord knows, there is always plenty of buzzing in there.

With Zen running, you are supposed to focus on breathing, your feet as they strike the ground, how the body feels, and the sights, sounds, and smells of nature. It's important not to think about the past or the future but remain in the moment. I found this difficult at first, but once I got the hang of it, the whole world melted away.

Even if it was only while out on the road.

The contemplation part is actually much easier than the concentrating. I use running as a quiet interlude to think about what is important to me.

That beeping noise is really distracting. Doesn't it bother anyone else out here?

I try both of the concepts whenever I train at the beach. Sometimes I run on the boardwalk with my eyes closed, feeling my way along the road. It's fun but can be a little challenging. I once tripped over a homeless man. It was early, and he wasn't up yet. I'm pretty sure he didn't notice.

"Lisa? Lisa! Come on, Lisa!"

Who's yelling my name? Where is that coming from? Why don't they leave me alone? I want to clear my mind and run. Nothing but the road and me.

"Honey? You in there? Honey?"

Is that my husband? Where is he? I don't understand what's happening.

Is there a problem with my children?

I have to finish my run. I'm supposed to put in some strong mileage today. Why is he calling me? He sounds so worried, almost desperate. What's the matter?

"She's barely breathing. Her oxygenation level is dangerously low. If we can't reach her soon, we will have to intubate. Do you remember talking about that? It's when we put a tube down her throat and help her breathe with a ventilator."

God, I hate those things. I'm terrified of them, actually. I was visiting a friend in the ICU once, and a patient in the bed next to her had one. It was horrible. He'd had a stroke that left him completely incapacitated. He couldn't do anything for himself, not even breathe or eat. The only organs that functioned properly were his heart and brain. He was fully conscious and could feel everything. The poor man had been there for over a week before the staff realized he had felt the surgical procedure they had performed. The nurses finally got him some pain medication, although it could do nothing to relieve the agony he must have endured earlier.

There was no living will or family to say it was okay to pull the plug, so they were legally required to keep him alive. It was a nightmare to see; I can't imagine what a nightmare it was to live.

Ouch! What was that? That really hurt! What is going on here?

Oh, my God.

I'm not running at all. My worst nightmare has come true.

I'm just like that guy, locked inside my own body.

That annoying beeping was the sound of all the monitors hooked up to my lifeless frame. Why was I so unresponsive? What happened to me?

And where was I? I couldn't see anything but sensed everything. I heard people talking, but they seemed distant. Why couldn't I see them? Why couldn't I reach them?

Was I dead?

Gradually, my mind cleared.

I remembered struggling physically the previous few weeks. My body had deteriorated quickly after my appointment with the ocular neurologist. We'd tried to get in with the other neurologist he had recommended, but there was a four-month wait. I'd had trouble with the movement of my limbs all week and hadn't been able to eat or drink for a couple of days, because I couldn't swallow. The thing with myasthenia is that the brain can send a message to the muscles, but nobody is home to answer the door. So nothing moves. Even my diaphragm, which controls breathing, had stopped working.

My body had given up. It just stopped in the middle of the race. One day I was at the head of the pack. The next day, I was on the side of the street like road kill.

How did this happen?

Myasthenia gravis. A title I could barely pronounce only weeks before had taken control of everything. This vile autoimmune disease, which started with double vision, had turned into the horror movie I now lived with.

At first, I tried to pretend it wasn't an issue and kept living my life, determined not to the let MG win. But what's that saying? Whatever you resist persists? This challenge not only continued but built up some serious steam in the process. All too quickly, I'd landed in a sterile hospital room, surrounded by people I didn't know, all of them trying to keep me alive.

But why are they working so hard? Who would want to live like this?

I wasn't sure I could handle a body that had retreated into a shadow of what it once was. I'd been betrayed by my own flesh, which left me nothing but a motionless corpse. Gone were the possibilities of ever feeling the summer sun on my face, the anticipation of joyfully screaming children on Christmas morning, or the touch of my husband's hand against my bare skin.

Wait. My husband. Is that him holding my hand? Is that who's crying?
And what about my children? How can I leave them while they are so young?
Is a fraction of a mother better than no mother at all?

"Sixty over thirty-five and dropping!" I heard someone say. Could that be my blood pressure?

Should I stop fighting and hand my life over to this autoimmune beast that ravaged me? Or should I salvage what was left of my being and figure out what to do with it later?

I wasn't afraid of death anymore. In essence, I'd been living in both worlds since I'd taken a turn for the worse. Half the time, I wasn't sure which was real anyway. I simply floated through space. I heard the voices of those around me again, but they bounced through my head without really connecting to my thoughts. Maybe this was my moment to leave. I wondered if the world would be better off without me. After all, I wasn't much of a contributor anymore. Spending every day lying in bed, gasping for one more breath, didn't amount to much in the grand scheme.

Should I release the tether connecting me to this world?

I hated that ridiculously painful tube they wanted to shove down my esophagus. I'd had it during my cancer surgeries and knew if they put that thing in me again, I would have sores in my mouth and throat for weeks. I couldn't afford to lose any more weight either. I had already seen the pity in people's eyes when they looked at my frail frame.

Dear God, what do I do?

The life force was draining from my body. I started to let go of my place in the world. Then I heard that voice, strong yet gentle, as if whispering softly from another world.

"Why don't you stop resisting us and yourself and learn the lessons we are trying to teach you, Lisa?"

Who is that? Hello?

"I'm here. I've always been here. But you haven't been listening."

Man, that sounded like something my husband would say. Who are you?

"I am the part of you that is connected to all. I am the piece of your higher self that touches the hand of God. I am the little voice in you that was squelched so many years ago. We had to take some drastic measures to clear you of all your busyness so you could find us again. I am the possibility of who you could be."

Okay, what do I call you? And where are you?

"I am always with you. I am in your dreams, the whisper in a gentle breeze, the random song on the radio that rings true. I am all around you. You can call me Melville, if you want."

Melville? Seriously? Why Melville? It figures that I would end up with someone named Melville.

"Because that is what you are comfortable calling me at the moment. Besides, what's in a name? You have bigger issues to worry about. You are at a fork in the road, and you need to make a decision about which path to follow. I know how hard it has been lately, and your struggle and the fight have been noted. It's okay to release the fragile tie that barely holds you here; no one will think less of you. Or you can continue to battle. It won't be easy, and taking that route means digging deeper than you ever knew possible, but the rewards will be greater than expected, too. The decision is yours. Remember, though, that death is not failure; it's merely a transition. Choosing life will offer great rewards in wisdom, but there is always a cost. We will walk every step of the way with you, as we do with every soul that travels this planet, but you must choose."

I had to decide whether I wanted to live or die? I felt so tired. I'd fought for every breath I took for so long. My feeble body kept withering away until I feared there would soon be nothing left but dust. It would be so easy to let go, to stop the fight. I could be at peace in a matter of minutes, at one with my Creator.

So what was stopping me?

Then I remembered: I'd never taken the easy route, never, ever. It's just not who I am. Besides, I wasn't done. I still needed to learn so much. There were also those little lives at home that depended on me. They were waiting for their mommy to come home and love them again. I couldn't let them or my husband down.

Okay, here we go.

I want to stay. As hard as life has been lately, I'm not ready to say goodbye to it or my family yet. What do I need to do to live, Melville?

"This is the easy part. All you have to do is open your eyes. Besides, you are scaring your husband. We will talk again. Look for me, and I will be there."

You will be where?

"Look to your internal compass. It will point you to where you need to be. Let faith lead the way. Now, wake up!"

I remember gasping for air. It felt as if someone had opened the nozzle to let the flow of oxygen back into my lungs. I jetted up, almost falling off the gurney. My eyes opened to see looks of shock and bewilderment on the faces of the people standing around me as they jumped back.

"The steroids must have kicked in," someone said.

The resident holding the tube looked almost disappointed. "Maybe she was being a little overdramatic," he said, tossing the opened intubation kit in the trash. He must have won the coin toss from the other residents to insert it. The poor guy would have to return to the girl I'd heard vomiting in the room next door.

I knew better. It was my second chance. I had been given an opportunity to wipe the slate clean, to start fresh with a new perspective.

Finally, there was hope in my future. I just needed to find . . . who did I need to find again? Did I only imagine him? The vision was fading, like a vivid dream lost in the drone of a day.

What was his name again?

CHAPTER 11

If you are going through hell, keep going.
Winston Churchill

I LOOKED AT THE CHECK marks on the pad of paper next to me. It was now Day Ten in the Intensive Care Unit. I was starting to understand why prisoners track their time in incarceration; it helps keep them grounded in reality and kills a few hours in the process. After a while, the moments begin to melt into one another. You get weary from the sterility of the care in your continually weakened state and become numb to the process.

One evening I awoke (not that anyone could actually sleep in the ICU) to the manic screams of a man in the unit next to mine. Having pulled his IV and catheter out of his body, he decided to make a break for it. I saw him running half naked past my door, with security guards in hot pursuit. Secretly cheering him on, I prayed he would make it outside before the entry doors to the floor went on lockdown. Sadly, he was tackled and carried back to his room and tucked in. He did the same thing every night for the next week.

My nurse said bizarre behavior like that happens so often in the ICU that there is a medical term for it. It's called hospital psychosis. People can actually go crazy because they are in the hospital for too long. He explained that a hospital environment can be extremely stressful for patients, but I was already clear on that. The combination of noisy medical equipment, unfamiliar surroundings, and disorienting lighting can lead to hallucinations, confused speech, and memory loss. The ICU is a little like Las Vegas . . . it's loud and windowless, and the lights are continually on. He said he'd had a patient the previous week who thought the wallpaper was talking to her.

I was pretty sure I was going a little nuts, too. I desperately missed my family and my dog and really wanted to go home.

What was the point of staying? I wasn't getting any better. If this was as good as it got, I even wasn't sure I wanted to go on living.

The doctors were treating me with something called plasmapheresis, a purification system that involved removing my blood through a central line in my neck and running it through a centrifuge to replace the plasma with albumin, a protein typically made in the liver. The goal was to get rid of the antibodies in my blood that were slowly destroying me. It's sort of the modern version of medieval bloodletting. I had such a violent response from the procedure that I passed out each time, and my blood pressure dropped so low that it was almost untraceable.

I underwent this procedure every day for two weeks.

As the days rolled on, I felt my life force slowly draining from my body again. My sanity depended on the nightly visits from my husband, who could sense me slipping away, as well. Although he was still working full time, running our house, and parenting our three busy children, he never missed sitting with me in the evenings and holding my hand. He also never let me see any sign of the exhaustion or fear he must have felt.

After straightening my bed linens and holding my head up so I could have something to drink, he would whisper, "Wanna go on vacation?"

I closed my eyes and imagined myself anywhere but where I was at that moment. "Sure, where do you want to go tonight?"

"I think Italy. I'm picturing that lovely little place by the canal in Venice where we sat after the gondola dropped us off. Remember how wonderful it was last time? "

Suddenly the room filled with the sounds and smells of a romantic Roman holiday.

"What are we having for dinner?" I asked, my eyes still closed.

"Oh, dinner! What a feast! The pasta and the fresh grilled fish look unbelievably good. The waiter greeted us with such a warm welcome, too. Nothing like having the best bottle of wine waiting at our table! By the way, you look so beautiful in that white, flowing dress, with your hair down."

His voice was just above a hush but so sweet in my ear.

"Thank you. You look great tonight, too."

"Do you hear the band playing our wedding song in the background? We are dancing slowly as the soft breeze picks up the wonderful aromas of the restaurant. It's late, but the night is just now coming alive with tourists, and the local children are still playing street games in the warmth of the summer evening. Can you see them lit up by the full moon?"

"I see them! They are having so much fun. You want to join them? I love playing with the kids."

"You betcha. I'll race you there! When we are tired, we can go back to our hotel overlooking the canal. I heard the gondoliers singing earlier, and we can listen to them as we drift off to sleep."

God bless that man. Thanks to him, I was transported from the stark, depressing hospital to an exotic oasis overflowing with the sounds and scents of a life where only health and happiness exist.

We'd never actually been to Venice or anywhere out of the country, for that matter, but every night he sat by my side and took me somewhere magical in my mind's eye, where we could dance the hours away in drunken abandonment.

I silently thanked him for filling me with fictional memories of faraway places. I would probably never be well enough to visit any of them, but at least we could run away together in our fantasy world. He truly was the keeper of my sanity. My heart sank when he had to leave me and go home. As he placed a goodbye kiss on my forehead, I smiled bravely, trying not to think of facing another night of screaming, insanity, and death.

CHAPTER 12

*Over the years your bodies become walking autobiographies, telling friends
and strangers alike of the minor and major stresses of your lives.*
Marilyn Ferguson

I WOKE UP EVERY MORNING to start the same process all over again.
I was beginning to accept my new routine as a normal way of life:

> *4:30 am — Wake up to a blood draw*
> *5:00 am — Vitals check*
> *5:30 am — Resident makes sure I am still alive for reports*
> *6:00 am — Rounds with medical students*
> *6:30 am — My doctors start their parades*

Each day also included three meals of cold, tasteless, liquefied
food, and careful measurements of every bodily fluid known to man.

I wondered how many others were staring at bare, depressing
hospital walls. And how many more were at home in their own beds
and doing the same? I've read that approximately fifty million
Americans or 20 percent of our population suffer from autoimmune
diseases. Fifty million aunts and grandpas, sisters and friends stand
alone in their fight for survival. Cancer has its battle cries. We grow
mustaches in November for prostate cancer, walk for days in
September for breast cancer, and buy daffodils in April to give to
those suffering from that dreaded disease.

Unfortunately, the term *autoimmune disease* is a catch-all phrase
for more than eighty "orphan" diseases looking for a home. Those

with autoimmune diseases are less organized because we do not recognize ourselves in each other. MG doesn't present its symptoms the way diseases like diabetes do, but the repercussions are no different. We pretend as long as we can that nothing is wrong, because ours is a communal problem that we don't fully understand. Autoimmune disease is the elephant in the room, sucking out the air (and our insurance dollars). It is the biggest unacknowledged issue we have in the medical arena.

Seventy-five percent of those affected are women just like me. That's thirty million women in our neighborhoods struggling to get their kids off to school in the morning because they are already too tired or physically limited in what they can do. As I lie here in my solitude, I think about how life used to be when I launched into each day with boundless energy. Now I need to lie down after I've brushed my teeth. I'm one of the lucky ones, as I have a husband who can cover us financially. What about all the single moms trying to navigate their own health issues alone while still putting food on the table for their families? To them, staring off into space is probably a luxury.

Men have it no better. I watched a dear friend of ours as his autoimmune disease viciously tore at his organs until there was nothing left. During the last year of his life, his family watched helplessly as this gentle giant crumbled into dust. I wonder what he was thinking as he stared at his own bare walls. Did he contemplate his existence, as I do? Did he feel as alone and powerless as I feel? My guess is that men probably feel more guilt and shame, because they are supposed to be the strong, dependable person in the family. As if there were any control over getting sick.

When there are multiple malfunctions in your body, you get to see lots of specialists. Pretty much anyone could come into my room and introduce himself as Doctor Blah-Blah from the blah-blah specialty, and I would automatically take my gown off. One would hope all of them were legit, but after a while I stopped caring. I never knew who was going to pop by, and that morning was no different.

The multitude of people in white coats typically shuffled through various updates on my condition, looking frantically for clues as to why I wasn't responding to . . . well . . . anything. They bellowed orders to my nurses, checked the computers hooked to various regions of my body, scribbled notes, and left. Occasionally, one would look at me to make sure there was an actual body in the bed. The usual suspects droned through that morning's rounds, with the exception of one bright, shiny new face.

"Hello, beautiful woman! How are you today?" He had a smile like sunshine and a face that lit up like an angel's.

I figured he was in the wrong room and probably the wrong hospital, too. "Who are you looking for?"

"You, of course, silly. I'm Dr. Habib. I am the integrative medicine doctor assigned to your case."

"I didn't know I had an integrative medicine doctor. What is an integrative medicine doctor?"

"I am a medical doctor, but I also use other modalities to treat the whole patient, not just the parts each doctor specializes in. My job is to help you bring your body back to balance."

"That's good, because Lord knows I'm seriously out of balance."

Dr. Habib was small in stature but large in energy. He seemed to float across the floor effortlessly before he sat down next to the bed and put his hand on mine. Gazing at me with incredible compassion, he lowered his voice and looked deeply into my eyes. "Dear girl, can you tell me why your chart has you listed as Do Not Resuscitate? Why are you giving up on yourself? Do you no longer want to live?"

I bowed my head in defeat, trying not to reveal my tear-stained face. With a voice ravaged by tubes and disease, my raspy whisper tried to explain. "It's just so hopeless. I keep getting worse, and nobody seems to know how to fix me. Every night, I lie in bed ready to go to sleep and wonder if I am going to wake up the next day. I have to fight for every breath I take. I choke on every ounce of liquid I try to swallow. I can't even remember the last time I ate solid food. I'm emaciated and exhausted. If this is the best it gets for me, I'm starting to wonder what I am fighting so hard for. If I stop breathing again, what kind of quality of life would I come back to?" I could no longer conceal the waterworks streaming down my contorted face. "I'm so tired of suffering."

I looked up and saw tears in his eyes, as well. "My dear girl, we are here as your guides to help you find your way, whichever road you choose. But, ultimately, you are responsible for your own destiny.

Huh?

Wow, was I confused. I'd never heard anything like that come from anyone in the medical profession. His statement momentarily snapped me out of my pity party.

"What do you mean? I don't know how to fix me."

"Sweet Lisa, there is nothing to fix, because you are not broken. Your body is in disharmony. Your beautiful instrument is out of sync, but with some proper tuning, you will one day be able to play beautiful music again. You are tired because you are fighting and denying your truth. You may not be the typical patient, but my sense is that you never were. This is probably why none of the normal protocols are working on you. Here is a little secret: there is no such thing as typical. We all have our own paths on our journeys in life. Maybe it is time to embrace yours and surrender to the situation you are in."

For the first time in a very long time, I felt an ounce of hope stream into my being. I wasn't sure why, since he hadn't given me anything tangible to indicate my situation would change, but I heard his words not only with my ears but in my heart, too. As frail as I was, I started to feel something I hadn't for years: empowered.

"How do I do that?"

"We need to start from the bottom up, to go deep to the ground floor and rebuild from the foundation, starting on the cellular level. Your recreation needs to be all-encompassing, involving your mind, body, and soul."

That sounded like a lot of work.

"I'm so weak I can't even get out of this bed without assistance. I can barely lift my arms, let alone walk. Where am I going to find the strength to do all this?"

"When I look in your eyes, I see the power of a warrior and the heart of a healer. You have all the tools you need already; you just have to remember how to use them. I will be here, as well, to assist you in the process. You can use Western medicine, in addition to other methods, to soothe, calm, and reenergize your systems. It's time to stop fighting and start working with the lessons you are here to learn from this process. You can do this. You are a true warrior; I know it from the strong pulse I feel in your wrist."

"Stop fighting? I thought fighting was what everyone wanted me to do. If I stop fighting back, isn't that giving in to this disease and letting it win?"

Dr. Habib leaned back in his chair and closed his eyes. His comfort with the unnaturally long period of silence that followed made me uneasy. Finally, he sat forward as if he had found the proper story in his mental index.

"There is a difference between giving in and leaning in. Sometimes it's not what is happening but how you handle it that dictates the final result. A parable is told of a farmer who owned an old mule. The mule fell into the farmer's well. The farmer heard the mule braying . . . or whatever mules do when they fall into wells. Although the farmer sympathized with the mule, after carefully assessing the situation, he decided that neither the mule nor the well was worth the trouble of saving. Instead, he called his neighbors together and told them what had happened. He then enlisted them to help him haul dirt to bury the old mule in the well and put him out of his misery.

The mule became hysterical as soil was repeatedly tossed into the well. But while the farmer and his neighbors continued shoveling, he realized that every time a load of dirt landed on his back, he could shake it off and step up on the growing mound of soil planted firmly beneath his feet. This he did, blow after blow.

Shake it off and step up. Shake it off and step up. Shake it off and step up. He repeated the encouragement to himself. No matter how painful the blows or how distressing his dilemma, the old mule fought the urge to panic and kept right on shaking off the dirt and stepping up.

It wasn't long before the mule, battered and exhausted, stepped triumphantly over the wall of that well! What was intended to bury him had blessed him . . . all due to the manner in which he had handled his adversity."

The doctor sat back in his chair again. Another awkward pause filled the room as he contemplated the story. Finally, I broke the silence.

"So, you think I'm the mule? I am battered and exhausted like the mule. I'm also as stubborn as the mule."

"You can be all of those things if you choose to be. Or none of them. Or you can be mule-like and lean into your struggles, letting them flow through you instead of resisting or fighting them."

"If I lean into them, will they go away?"

"Unfortunately, it isn't that easy. However, life is never one-dimensional either. If we face our problems and respond to them positively, refusing to surrender to bitterness or self-pity, the adversities that come along to bury us usually carry within them the potential to benefit and bless us."

Smiling, he stood and floated out the door again.

I felt as if I had been visited by divine intervention. I wasn't sure how that man had wandered into my room, but I was very happy he had. My mind was spinning from our conversation and filled with questions, anticipation, and, for the first time since my diagnosis, faith that I could make it through to the other side.

I find it fascinating that a random person can pop into your life, drop a few pearls of wisdom, and change your perspective forever. It makes me wonder if there really are angels sent from God, roaming the planet to heal our hurts. If that is true, I was sure this little guy was one of them. I believe we all meet these people from time to time; we just don't always recognize them. Looking back, I can still visualize some of mine: the homeless guy who told me how pretty I looked when I felt like Medusa, the stranger who ran to drop money in my meter before I got a ticket, and even the dog in the park that licked my hand after sensing my sadness when mine had died. How many other angels had come to help when I was too busy to see? It reminded me of a song from my youth. I think the words were "I once was lost and now am found. Was blind, but now I see."

Now that I have slowed down, I have vowed to always keep my eyes open. Grace really is amazing.

CHAPTER 13

FINALLY, DAY 14 ARRIVED.

I wasn't sure if surviving two weeks in the ICU should be viewed as a milestone or a miracle. Either way, it felt wonderful to finally be strong enough to transfer to a regular floor. The food tasted no better, but at least it made me optimistic that home might be around the corner, even if I had to be in a wheelchair until I regained my ability to walk again. I could also see out the small window across the room, which let me know whether it was day or night and gave me a view of the hospital roof and the employee parking garage below. For hours, I watched as the staff headed for their shifts, juggling packages, lunches, and cell phones as they mindlessly ran to their day at work.

Time had stopped for me, though. I felt like a ghost watching from a distant place as the living droned through their daily chores. Seeing the morning rush made me appreciate how many of us go through life unconsciously, unaware until it is too late. Even I had been walking this planet numb to all its beauty and precious gifts for way too long. As I sat perched in my sterile bed, looking out that window, I vowed never again to be just a voyeur.

Once free from these walls, I would be completely present in my life. I was determined to stop floating through it and actively participate in everything I did. I had made that promise to myself once before, after I finished my cancer treatments, but it didn't stick. This time would be different.

From my vantage point high above the busyness below, I wondered if part of me really had died in the ICU. It had to in order for the shell around my soul to finally crack. For a small, surreal moment that I hoped would last forever, I felt as if my breath connected me to every other breathing being on earth. As I watched the continual flow through the hallways, I sensed the collective heartbeat of humanity, as well, seeing through new eyes the dark and the light in myself and everyone around me. It was awe inspiring.

The connectedness to life overwhelmed me, and tears streamed down my pale face. I no longer felt totally alone in my pain and sadness or in my joy.

I also better understood what Dr. Habib meant when he spoke about taking ownership of my healing. I had begun to realize the anguish my soul must have felt when I shut out its voice long ago. I figured the emotional stress I constantly put myself under probably played a role in my illness, as well. I needed to stop being a victim of my circumstances and participate in my recovery. I may not have wanted this disease, but I had it in all its painful glory. I was ready to actively contribute to my recovery.

We all need to do our part and participate in our own healing, whether our illness is physical, emotional, or spiritual. Medicine can only do part of the work; the rest is up to us. The hospital stay had given me the gift of sustainable life, but it was up to me to finally live it. The time to do my own recreating had arrived, and I needed to clear out the debris in my mind, body, and soul to make space for a new consciousness. Things started to feel different in my body, as if my DNA was being activated for a different path from the one I had followed to that point.

I had no idea how to implement any of the thoughts running through my mind, nor did I fully understand them. However, I truly believed that if I set that desire as my intention, the teachers I needed would somehow manifest themselves to show me the way.

That night, a sense of peace washed over me as I drifted off to sleep after watching the sun set behind the air conditioning unit on the roof. Realizing I had spent almost the entire day looking out the window, I smiled to myself.

It took almost dying again to comprehend that I hadn't been living. Many would consider staring out a window a waste of time. In hindsight, I think the view helped me understand all I had missed by spending so many years looking but never seeing.

It made me wonder why we consume so much of our time on the trivial when there is so much more out there that warrants our attention.

CHAPTER 14

Tell your heart that the fear of suffering is worse than the suffering itself.
Paulo Coelho

AFTER MY FIRST COUPLE of rounds with cancer, I remember telling someone at church about my medical history. As I rattled off facts related to my various health issues, she looked at me with eyes filled with horror.

Then she asked me how it felt to be ignored by God. I wasn't sure I understood the question.

The well-meaning woman then pulled out her Bible and read a passage. "Ask and it will be given to you; seek and you will find; knock and the door will be opened to you." She said God hadn't healed me because I probably wasn't praying hard enough for an end to my suffering. She asked if I wanted to pray with her for God to fix all the broken pieces of my life.

Was my life that broken? I'd thought it was my body that was a mess. Was there more I needed to fix?

The woman continued by telling me a story about a friend of hers whose cancer was so devastating that all the doctors could offer was the removal of every organ below her waist, replacing them with tubes and bags. The night before the surgery, the woman's minister organized a vigil to lay hands on her and pray. During routine surgical prep the next day, the physician did a scan to map out the diseased organs. To his amazement, the cancer had completely disappeared. The woman was inexplicably healed.

The point the church lady was trying to make was that God can deliver us from any unfortunate situation if we pray hard enough and if it is His will to do so.

Did she really think that I was still sick because I hadn't been praying enough? I assured her that wasn't the case.

In that event, she said, either I had done something wrong and illness was my penance or God didn't want me to be healed. Since I'd been praying for healing, she was curious how I felt about God's rejection.

I was speechless.

Why do people assume that not getting their way means God has disregarded them or is mad? Is it our job to manipulate God?

Is that even possible?

And why do folks feel the need to tell those with serious illnesses about friends and relatives who were restored miraculously?

I am thrilled for them, of course, but after countless surgeries, debilitating chemo, and painful radiation, I don't really want to hear about the people who got to skip to the front of the line because they were favored by God. It makes me feel bad.

Did that woman really believe He was mad at me?

Why do we assume when our desires don't arrive within our time frame that something has to be wrong? Maybe God is just saying, "Not right now" or "Hang tight, because I have something else in mind for you."

My daughter listens to a Garth Brooks song titled "Thank God for Unanswered Prayers." Maybe Garth was onto something.

Sometimes, our lessons come easily; other times, not so much. Don't get me wrong. If someone were to offer illness as a learning method, I would pass it up in a heartbeat. Once on our trajectory, however, we may as well accept the ride as gracefully as possible and hopefully gain a little wisdom along the way.

Unanswered prayers are often our biggest opportunities for growth. Even with the hardships that are involved, they may arrive with many blessings, too, if we look hard enough.

My husband says we are founding members of the two-by-four club. It means God has to hit us over the head with a piece of wood to get our attention, because we are either too dense or too stubborn to learn anything from books or other people's trials. Although there are much less painful ways to study, experience seems to be the only way for me to truly get the intended lessons.

It's unfortunate, but I think the harder way of learning is more common for most of us. I know that has always been the case for me.

I don't believe God ignores us at all. Instead, He walks with us through our trials while holding our hands and helping us navigate the darkness. He isn't saying, "No, Lisa, I am going to let you and your family suffer unbelievable pain, because I am busy elsewhere, and you haven't been to church enough anyway." Instead, I think he is telling me, "Look, this is really going to suck, but I will be walking through the valley with you. When it is over, we will be closer than ever, and you will be wiser for it."

God's school of hard knocks may not be painless, but it is very effective.

If we have to go through trials we don't enjoy, why not stop blaming God for not doing his job properly and glean all we can from every experience by letting Him teach?

When life circles around and around the same issue, like vultures hunting their prey, we should probably take a beat and ask why this is happening.

I made a decision to stop viewing my health as simply another hardship I had to endure and go deeper by looking for the reason why illness was becoming a repetitive theme in my life. It wasn't enough to find the right balance of medications. I wanted to use this disease as a catalyst to further my growth and search for answers to questions I had not yet formed.

Someone once told me that the five stages of grief are denial, anger, bargaining, depression, and acceptance. I think that is true when dealing with serious illnesses, as well. I had tried denying I was sick, and I almost ended up in a very bad car accident. Anger alienated me from those I loved most, since they are usually the ones we lash out at the hardest. Bargaining hadn't worked, and I was tired of being depressed. I needed to accept that God wasn't going to deliver me from anything the easy way. I had to figure out what my family and I were to learn while finding some sort of joy in the process. It would be no easy feat but better than the despair I was barely keeping at bay.

I would never encourage anyone to actively seek life-threatening situations, but if they happen, you may begin to see life from a much broader frame of reference. You may also realize there is more strength in each of us than we realize.

My next move was to stretch farther than I believed possible. To reach beyond my limits and look at myself not as broken (as the church lady had suggested) but as changing or morphing from what once was to what could be.

All I needed was a little help. Or maybe a lot of help.

MIND

CHAPTER 15

Change is not a matter of possibility; it's a matter of decision.
Kevin Ngo

FINALLY OUT OF THE HOSPITAL and feeling a little stronger, I found myself back in the normal routine of sitting in various medical offices for my regular checkups. I thought about how much time I spent waiting for doctors and wondered how far they would get in the business world if they made their clients wait two or three hours for every appointment. This particular specialist, of course, wasn't the only practitioner in my life to triple book appointments. Maybe instead of offering five-year-old entertainment magazines to keep us occupied, they should install kiosks with online college courses to help us further our education. Given the amount of time I'd spent sitting around, I could have become a physician myself and found a cure for all our diseases by now.

After being escorted to the freezing exam room, I waited another 45 minutes in my paper gown, shivering. The doctor came in with his usual stack of folders and a grumpy disposition.

"I have the results of your test here somewhere," he snarled without looking up to greet me.

"And did I pass?" I was attempting a little humor to lighten him up. I can usually warm up anyone, but I was starting to suspect the room wasn't cold just because the thermostat was set to fifty degrees.

"What?" He looked a little annoyed that I had spoken to him.

"Never mind. What do they say?"

"Oh. We ran a few more tests while you were in the hospital.

Along with the myasthenia gravis, you now test positive for lupus, another autoimmune disease. That's probably part of the reason you weren't responding to the treatments very well. You were taking your own sweet time getting out of the ICU, for sure."

The intercom buzzed. "Sir, you have a call on line one."

"I'll be back in a minute," he snapped. Then he whirled around and walked out of the door faster than I'd seen him move before.

Have you ever wondered why someone so incredibly bad with people would want to work in a field that actually involves interacting with people?

Almost half an hour went by before I popped my head out of the door. No physician in sight. After another twenty minutes, a nurse came in and looked startled to see me.

"Oh, you're still here?"

"Yes, I was waiting for the doctor to finish our meeting." That statement didn't come out fluidly, because I was so cold my lips were blue and practically immobile.

"Sorry, dear. He had an emergency and left for the hospital. You will have to reschedule."

"Okay. Thanks."

In my mind, I was furious. I'd wasted an entire afternoon I would never get back, waiting for a man who dropped a bomb on me and walked out the door. He was the same guy who wanted me to get a psych evaluation when I first got sick, because he thought I was faking it. I wondered if I should have my sanity checked, after all, for keeping him on my medical team.

That got me thinking. Why was I willing to patiently wait for hours for a doctor who had no bedside manner, allow him to blow up my world by delivering horrible news, and then calmly watch him leave?

Why did people treat me that way?

I think I have the answer to that question. Because I allowed it to happen.

Too often, we let others do their thing without voicing an objection. I felt as if years of anger and resentment had built up inside my body. I didn't speak up for fear of hurting someone else's feelings. Maybe I should start caring more about my own.

In that moment of clarity, I realized something. There is a theory that unprocessed stress accumulates in the body. Eventually, it causes enough damage that a physical manifestation of all that stress appears, like getting a stomach ulcer from too much anxiety. Thyroid and thymus cancer, chronic childhood tonsillitis, and strep throat, all issues I have had, start in the throat. Could bottled-up anger have been sitting in that area until it finally caused a serious medical malfunction? I couldn't imagine anger-fueled stress as the total cause, but it certainly might have contributed to my health problems. It was worth looking into.

I had wasted too much time watching my life from the sidelines without being my own referee. Silent Lisa was leaving that facility never to return, physically and metaphorically. I didn't intend to become a raging lunatic, screaming about every wrongdoing, but it was finally my chance to speak up and speak my truth.

We all have to speak our truth.

Why are we so afraid to have a voice in this world, especially when it comes to those we deem better than ourselves-like medical professionals? No one is truly higher or lower. Hierarchy is just a state of mind.

And I was starting to mind.

The label "patient" does not translate to "low man on the totem pole." It just means we need a little help getting back to balanced health.

If he wasn't going to help me, then I was ready to find someone who would. Someone who would see me as a person, not just an interesting case.

CHAPTER 16

I WENT HOME AND STARTED my Internet search on lupus, since I had no idea what it was or how it would affect me.

Then my neighbor Maude called.

I barely had time to say hello before she started her rant. "Oh, my God! You wouldn't believe what happened to me this morning. I was in line at The Coffee Bean, and this man came up and stood right in front of me. I told him that the end of the line was out the door, and he had the nerve to tell me he was in a hurry and couldn't wait. So he thought it was okay to cut in line! Can you believe that? I said, 'Look Buddy, I'm waiting, and all of these other people are waiting, and you are going to have to wait, too.' He got mad at me, but I just turned around and got mad right back at him. Can you imagine?"

No, I couldn't imagine at all.

At first I was a little annoyed by her story. Didn't she realize I was trying to research lupus, since my doctor hadn't bothered to explain it before he left me alone in a freezing room, wearing nothing but a paper gown?

Wait. The answer was no, she didn't know. I hadn't told her.

Wouldn't it be interesting if that rude man in the coffee shop had been my obnoxious endocrinologist?

As self-absorbed as Maude can be, she doesn't let anyone or anything trample over her. She stands up for herself. I'll bet her throat area is completely disease free.

When I grow up, maybe I should be more like my friend.

"I'm sorry that happened to you, Maude. I found out this morning that I tested positive for lupus on top of all my other health issues, and I have no idea what that means. I have to go so I can read up on it."

Just like that, I said something.

I rather enjoyed saying something. If that was how it felt to have a voice, I might have to speak up more often.

Usually, I would be on the phone another half hour without speaking, listening to her ramble, but I had had enough. I didn't care if she was upset; I needed to move on with my information search.

For a moment, there was nothing but silence on the other end of the phone. Then she spoke. "Lupus? Wow. That's awful. How do you feel about it?"

A wave of emotion suddenly overpowered me, like the tsunami I so often dreamt about. "Honestly, I feel as if I am being held together with duct tape and chicken wire these days. I could unravel at any moment."

She slowed her speech, speaking softly. "You know, my cousin has lupus. She goes to a great doctor, if you want her number. The office is not very far from you."

Had Maude really focused on me and my needs? And even asked how I was feeling? That hadn't happened before. We didn't do feelings. At least we hadn't until then.

"Thanks for listening, Maude, and for your help. It would be great to get the number. I think it's time to find another doctor."

It was time to move forward on many levels of my life.

It was also time to take some responsibility for my own actions and stop blaming others for ignoring me. My body began to relax almost immediately, as my throat felt less restricted for the first time. The mere thought of saying my piece gave me peace. Who knew it would be so easy? Speaking what was on my mind had always been a terrifying concept, but I saw it then as part of the healing process for my body.

I thought about the notes in the dream journal I'd kept in the hospital. What was it I'd written? *Small changes in behavior equal cataclysmic results.*

Looking back, I don't remember why I wrote that or what context it came from, but maybe this was one of the baby steps necessary to take charge of my life and begin to return my health to balance.

As I looked out my window, a hummingbird buzzed by. I heard myself saying, "Do you think unprocessed emotional issues contributed to my medical meltdown?"

I wasn't sure why I felt the need to speak with a hummingbird. I was pretty certain the solution I sought didn't rest with him.

Even though I couldn't answer my question either, it was worth some investigation.

The more pressing question was how?

CHAPTER 17

Be who you are and say what you feel, because those who mind don't matter and those who matter don't mind.

Dr. Seuss

LIKE MANY PROCRASTINATORS, when I am at a loss as to what to do, I avoid making any decision at all until absolutely forced to do so. Since that habit hasn't served me well historically, I thought I would try something different. Having limited resources for changing my journey's trajectory, I decided to start by asking the friends I meet with weekly; we call ourselves the Coffee Club.

I first met these women many years ago when we bought our starter homes in our starter neighborhood at about the same time. The term "starter" is code for cheap, small homes built on an old cow pasture. Our children were around the same age, as well. With our husbands distracted by their respective careers, we bonded together, trying to figure out motherhood and who we were supposed to be in the world. After a few years had passed, it became clear that although we lived on the same block, our lives had not necessarily traveled the same street. As I slowly withdrew from my social circle due to ongoing health issues, my neighbors meandered along other paths.

Eventually, our lack of common interests made it uncomfortable to be together for extended periods. Predominately to stay off each other's nerves, we lovingly limited our social interaction to coffee on Tuesday mornings. Thus, the title "Coffee Club."

Our meetings typically started with a few anecdotes about our husbands or children, followed by tidbits about what was on sale and where. Then we jumped into anything else we could think of to kill the rest of the hour.

That morning, I decided to change the normal routine by jumping right into the deeper matters that were on my mind. It wasn't that I considered the Coffee Club a particularly safe environment in which to speak from the heart, but I was desperate and had nowhere else to turn. How bad could it be? The worst they could do was kick me out of the group and talk about me behind my back. I was pretty sure they'd already done the talking-behind-my-back part anyway.

Although I don't play golf, I'm fond of a golf expression my husband uses: Never up, never in. I like the fearless connotation and find the questioning looks when using the term amusing. Taking a deep breath, I went all in by saying, "I was thinking about going to a therapist to see if there is an emotional component to my physical disease. Have any of you ever gone to one?"

It was like diving into the shallow end of the pool head first. The initial response was from Maude. It was not very favorable.

"Good God! Therapy? Seriously, Lisa, that is for women with too much free time on their hands." Maude paused to pour several flasks of "herbal tonic" into her latte. "Why on earth do you need therapy? Oh, are you having marital problems? Did you find drugs in one of your kid's rooms? Wait . . . that was Allison down the street who found pot in her son's closet. Did I tell you what my Mike did the other day at school?"

And off we went to the world of Maude.

The best thing about having narcissistic friends is that you never have to worry about what you will be talking about. As long as the conversation cycles back to them, that is.

After she was done with her gossip about . . . whatever it was . . . I threw the question out there again.

"Have any of the rest of you ever tried therapy?"

Minnie's weary eyes filled with tears.

"What's wrong, Minnie?" I asked, already knowing the answer.

She sat back in her chair and clutched her tea with closed eyes. "I was trying to picture myself in a space all my own, where I could work on me and my issues, a place that doesn't include a baby attached to my breast, sucking the energy out of me, or someone calling my name so I can help them do something. I haven't slept in five years. I'm so physically and emotionally drained, and everyone takes a piece of me until there is nothing else to give. If I had a minute to look at myself and my life, I would probably head to the grocery store for milk and never go back."

Before I could respond to her cry for help, a familiar, high-pitched voice to my left chimed in. "Why would anyone spend all that time and money talking about things you can't change . . . or that you'd really prefer to forget . . . when you can medicate? Wait! You never answered Maude. Is your husband cheating on you? If that's the case, you don't have to worry about a therapist, because I have a great lawyer. He will take him for everything he has!" Cheryl was perfectly serious. "You know, ever since my doctor put me on Paxil, I'm perfectly Zen. And with my new attorney taking over the divorce, I'll have plenty of money to pay for it, too," she said with a chuckle.

"I'll drink to that!" Maude said, lifting her latte in salute.

Cheryl's husband had announced not long before that he was leaving her for a man and had only used her to help pay the tuition for his school.

It was a lot for her to process.

I wondered how much of Cheryl's day was Zen and how much of it was spent escaping her pain by numbing herself with prescription drugs. Unfortunately, she was also numbing the rest of her personality. When we talked, she never seemed fully present. She'd been through a lot emotionally, and her coping method seemed to be working for her in the short term, but I wondered how well it would work in the long run. On the other hand, Cheryl didn't have to deal with checking into the hospital every six months due to a life-threatening illness. My motivation was different. If I didn't climb on top of things soon, I feared my stupid disease would end up killing me.

From across the table, Gabby added, "I think there are lots of ways to deal with problems. I like zoning out when I'm stressed. I typically turn on the TV and channel surf, especially during the day. Sometimes, it's fun to watch one of those reality shows where everyone is drunk and fighting. Once I'm tired of watching TV, I go shopping or spend a couple of hours on the computer. It always makes me feel better."

And there it was. How Americans deal with their problems . . . or don't. It's no wonder we become more and more disconnected from ourselves and each other—we live in a "numb the pain" society. Spacing out in front of the TV while we watch mind-numbing shows, surfing the Internet, medicating (or self-medicating) ourselves, or simply droning through our existence seem to be the standard methods for coping with our problems these days.

There must be a better way.

There had to be a way to check in with myself and learn if my emotions really were affecting my physical body. But how? It had taken another knock on death's door to wake me up, but I had finally focused on figuring myself out. Working through any unresolved issues wasn't really a luxury for me. I needed to recreate a totally different me from the ground up, physically, emotionally, and spiritually.

After we all left the coffee shop, Gabby stopped me in the parking lot. She kept looking over her shoulder as if we were being followed and whispered, "You know, if you are really going to pursue this whole counseling thing, I know a guy. Actually, it's a woman. A friend had some luck with seeing her."

It felt like I was making a back-alley drug score instead of acquiring the phone number of someone who could possibly help me figure some things out. I decided to play along.

"Really, Gabby? What happened with your friend?"

"Oh, she was going through some things and needed some help; nothing big. I mean, her life was really great; she just needed to look at something small, and this lady helped her. You want her name and number?"

"Sure." I had no idea who else to call or where to go for a referral, so I figured a phone number from a friend's friend was better than nothing.

She looked around again to see if anyone was watching us. "Okay, but you didn't get it from me. And don't bring up my name if you call. Not that she would know me, but let's keep this between us."

"Your secret's safe with me, Gabby. I mean your friend's secret."

Why would admitting you need a little help from time to time be a secret? Are we so afraid to concede that we don't know everything and aren't perfect? I think it is pretty obvious to everyone else around us that we may have some problems here and there. Besides, no one teaches us how to process our feelings when we are growing up. Hell, it's hard for most of us to admit we even have feelings at all.

"Her name is Mona. She works on the west side of town, but she can do sessions by phone, too, which may be good for you since you can't drive very far. I should warn you, though, that it can be hard to schedule an appointment. I heard her waiting list is about six months long. Maybe, since you are sick, she can fit you in sooner."

Gabby certainly knew a lot of information about a woman she'd only heard about from a friend, but I wasn't going to mention that.

"Thanks. I will call her and let you know what happens."

She looked horrified. "No! I mean, that is private information. You don't have to share that with me . . . or anyone . . . ever. Why would you talk about stuff like personal issues or past traumas with us?" She looked genuinely puzzled.

"Because you all are my friends?" That would probably be an obvious answer for most groups but clearly not our group. Maybe we should change that.

She laughed. "You're thinking about coming clean with these women? They will eat you alive! Then they will talk about you afterwards. Are you sure you're ready to deal with that?"

She had a point. The women in our club had many good qualities, but no one would ever describe them as open or compassionate. Did I really want to throw what I might learn to this group of friends and risk being verbally killed for being vulnerable, even if it could change the dynamic of my little tribe in the process?

Perhaps I should keep my mouth shut. Or would it be easier to switch to another group? Both were possibilities.

It reminded me of the fairy tale about the swan and the ducks, where one of them was criticized because she didn't fit in with her group. One day, everything changed when she realized she wasn't a duck at all but something different.

Maybe I was swimming in the wrong pond.

Or maybe I should not worry about it. I was jumping ahead of myself anyway. I wouldn't have anything to share with the Coffee Club unless I got an appointment with Mona, and there was no guarantee that would happen.

Maybe instead of listening to all the circle jerking that was going on in my head, I should go home and make a phone call.

There seemed to be a lot of *maybe's* in my world. Could it be a sign that change and, potentially, growth were around the corner? Is that how we know we are changing, when things don't fit as well as they did before? Or do they fit better? My mind was expanding far beyond what I thought my limits were, as if my cerebral universe had expanded.

During my last pregnancy, I really enjoyed dessert and hit Girl Scout Cookie month hard. After my daughter was born, I was still fifty pounds overweight. Fortunately, I had two dear friends who were in the same boat, and we started exercising together. Months passed, and I watched as the pounds melted off them while I still struggled to zip up my fat jeans. One day, to my horror, I realized I'd run my jeans through a cycle in the dryer, making them even tighter. My discovery occurred moments before I had to do my preschool pickup duty, and there was no time to find something else to wear. To my astonishment, the jeans not only fit but were a little loose!

Sometimes we don't see change until it hits us in the face. What's important is embracing our transformations with love and acceptance, no matter how big or small, celebrating as each change slips into the grand puzzle of life.

CHAPTER 18

AS SOON AS I GOT HOME, I reached for the phone. To my surprise, Mona herself answered...no gatekeeper to filter out the crazies. I guess in that line of work, crazy is probably pretty commonplace. Her voice was soft and very calming, but I got stage fright as soon as I heard her speak.

"Uh, hello. This is Lisa. Is this Mona?"

What a stupid way to start a conversation. Thankfully, she ignored my greeting and introduced herself, asking how she could help me.

Before I could answer, my mind engaged in a conversation of its own.

How can she help me? Great question. I have no idea if she can, or if I even want her to. Wait, I'm the one who came up with the idea of trying therapy, so why am I choking on what to say next? Maybe I'm not ready to uncover my problems. Or maybe I already know what they are and am not ready to face them. Perhaps I'm afraid to look into my mind and see what lives there. Maybe I should stop talking to myself and just commit by making an appointment already. Or not.

I think they call that sort of mental conversation "spinning out of control." Perhaps the therapy thing was a pretty good idea for me after all.

I assumed that her schedule was full, so I decided to play a little game with myself. If she couldn't see me right away, I would look for another way to figure out if there was an emotional component involved in my getting sick. If she could fit me in, I would start right away.

I took a deep breath and rolled the dice. "I was wondering if you had any openings for new clients. I'm sure you're busy, but I have some medical issues and was wondering if there is more than the physical element that I should look at."

She paused for a second before speaking. "Well, let me look. I have been working with a client who is traveling overseas for a while, and her slot recently opened up. You busy next Thursday?"

Mild panic set in again. I wasn't sure why, but I sensed it welling up in my throat. With school out, the kids were at home, and I would have to arrange child care. Playing another game with myself, one that my husband calls mental masturbation, I decided that if I could get a babysitter, which was next to impossible on short notice, I would go. If not, I would pass on the appointment.

All those mind games made me start doubting that I was ready to commit to therapy. I told Mona my childcare situation and said I would have to call her back to confirm.

"Sure, honey. Your fate is up to you and you alone. Let me know how it goes."

What did she mean by that? Could she tell what was going on in my head? Was she aware that I was trying to find a way out so I wouldn't have to look at my dark side or whatever it was I didn't care to see? Could she sense my sudden fear through the phone?

She could surely sense the neurosis that was at play; it was a no brainer.

I chuckled out loud at the myriad of thoughts that had made themselves at home in my brain.

My next call was to my mother to see if she could stay with the kids. I knew she delivered peanut butter and jelly sandwiches to the homeless on Thursdays, so she would probably say no. I didn't plan to tell her where I needed to go, because I didn't want her to feel bad about her daughter needing mental help. I would hate for her to think she'd been a bad mother. After all, this wasn't about her. It was about me.

When she answered the phone, I asked the question, anticipating her scheduling conflict with relief. "Mom, can you watch the kids Thursday?"

She replied without hesitation. "Sure."

Oh.

"But don't you have sandwiches to deliver?"

"Nope."

Bummer.

"But you've been doing that for years."

"Exactly. I decided to give myself a little break. Father Mike is taking over for a couple of months starting this week, so I'm free on Thursdays now."

Damn.

It seemed I would have to face my issues after all.

I continued. "I might be busy every Thursday for a while. Would you be able to watch them every week?"

"Sure. I love spending time with my grandchildren."

"Don't you want to know what I'll be doing?"

"I don't care. Take some time for yourself."

She always cares about what I'm doing. How could she not care this time? Doesn't she love me anymore?

After listening to the chatter in my mind, seeing a therapist was looking more and more like something I truly needed to do.

I called Mona again and blurted my news. "Thursday works great for me. Can't wait."

That wasn't true. I could wait. Then, again, I truly couldn't wait. Living with MG wasn't getting any easier.

"Great, honey! Talk to you then."

Nervously, I asked, "What will we be talking about? If I had a little heads-up, I could prepare."

Wow. That sounded ridiculous even to me.

I could feel her smiling through the phone. "Don't worry. This is a very safe environment. The dunk tank is gone now."

"The what?"

"I had a tank in my office. You know, the big tubs of water where you sit on a ledge and wait to get dunked? If a client said the wrong thing, I threw a ball at the lever, and she got dumped in. It was a real ice breaker."

I was sweating. "Seriously?"

"No. Of course not, silly. I'm messing with you."

Did I need a therapist who could mess with my mind more than I did? Maybe.

"So I take it you won't tell me what we will be doing."

"How can I tell you when I have no idea? We'll find out together."

"I don't think I have too many issues, but I keep getting sick. Very sick. And I'm starting to think there is an emotional connection. I figure if people with too much anxiety get ulcers and stress can bring on hives, then I must have some serious problems."

"If you are on this planet, you have issues. It's how we learn and grow. Learning how to process through them is where the wisdom happens. No matter how much you think you understand about processing your feelings, there is always room for growth and more to understand about how they affect your entire life. It's like skinning an onion, honey. No matter how many layers you peel away, there is always another one to remove. It's simply a matter of how deep you're ready to go."

My eyes welled up with tears as I started to sniffle.

"Why are you crying, sweetie?" she asked softly.

"I have no idea. Do you?"

Her tone became even sweeter. "Maybe deep inside my words are ringing true in your heart. You already have all the answers you need. You just have to remember them."

I think she was overestimating me and my ability to comprehend what she was referring to.

"What if I look and find more than I can handle? I've never met anyone else who has had three different types of cancer and two autoimmune diseases at my age . . . or any age, for that matter. Six friends who had only a few of the things I've had are dead now. They are all gone, and I'm still here, and I don't understand why."

"Do you know what that makes you?"

"Stubborn? Stupid?" I was pretty sure it was one of those.

"How about strong and determined to get whatever lesson you are here to learn."

Her interpretation sounded better than mine.

"I would like to get this. I just can't figure out what *this* is."

She laughed. "Well, let's find out together! Discover the struggle, learn the lesson, know the purpose. It's a Monaism."

"What's a Monaism?"

"Little sayings I came up with that help folks remember my teachings."

"Mona proverbs?"

"Exactly. Talk to you later, punkin!"

I had a feeling I was going to like her. Anyone who pretends she has a dunk tank and comes up with her own proverbs could be fun to work with.

I was excited to see where we could go together emotionally.

And terrified.

I seemed to be living in *terrified* much of the time. I was tired of always being so scared of life. Maybe that was something we could look at first.

CHAPTER 19

Consider the postage stamp: its usefulness consists in the ability to stick to one thing till it gets there.
Josh Billings

THURSDAY ARRIVED too quickly. I wasn't sure why I was still nervous about meeting Mona. Maybe it was because until then I had never seriously considered that I may have played a part in my own illness. Or was it because she'd been a bit intimidating on the phone with the dunk tank talk? Regardless, I felt uncomfortably transparent.

I couldn't believe my eyes when I walked in for my appointment. Halloween was a week away, and her office had been transformed into a haunted house, complete with skeletons offering both decapitation and candy. Mona herself wore a goblin costume.

Seriously? I'd finally decided to see a therapist, and she appeared to be crazier than me? What were the odds?

Pretty high, considering my luck. According to the law of attraction, we invite the people who are most like us into our lives. It's kind of a birds-of-a-feather concept, like in high school when all the jocks hang out in one corner, stoners in another, and brains in the lab. If the law applied to me in this situation, I was in more trouble than originally anticipated.

Hopefully, Mona provided a punch card where you pay for five sessions and get the sixth one free or some other type of frequent flyer plan. I might need it.

As I sat on the couch next to a life-sized vampire, all I could say was, "Wow, is Halloween your favorite holiday?"

She looked around absently. "No. I decorate like this for every holiday. You should see what I do to the place for Kwanza."

"You celebrate Kwanza?" I tried to remember what Kwanza was.

"I celebrate everything! We all should do more celebrating of life, don't you think?"

What I was really thinking was that I might need to rethink the therapy idea.

Describing Mona is almost impossible. She was a firecracker of energy packed in one compact blonde package . . . and very theatrical in a fun way. I imagine if Mona had to pick another body to live in, she would be an outrageously flamboyant gay man, considering that much of her daily wardrobe resembled Liberace's. Her career as a dancer on Broadway had ended abruptly many years before when she contracted an indefinable but life-threatening disease and ended up in a wheelchair. She learned to walk again and eventually ran a marathon.

A true study in contrasts, Mona had attended a remedial high school but frequently gave graduation speeches at prestigious colleges. She left her fundamentalist Christian husband to live with her girlfriend while raising her son and a few other children, as well. My new therapist was part brilliant, part totally nuts, part spiritual guru, and part little girl. Although kindhearted and understanding, the woman could also be tough as nails. She would read your mind, sense your heart, and kick your butt to the curb . . . all at the same time.

It took only a couple of sessions of getting to know each other before we went after the heavy stuff. Mona didn't mess around with anyone's time.

She made me question everything I thought I knew, but I kept returning for more. Her unconventional methods seemed to work, and I liked the changes I was starting to see in myself. In one of our first sessions, she helped me gain a new perspective on my illness. She said, "Whether we're dealing with myasthenia gravis, cancer, alcoholism, workaholism, eating disorders, or ego, we are all diseased. Your issue is just more definable, which isn't a bad thing. Others spend their whole lives sensing that something is not quite right in their world without ever understanding the problem. You can physically feel and see what you are dealing with and how it manifests on an emotional level."

I wasn't sure I totally agreed with what she was saying, but I was willing to go deeper. After a few months of studying with Mona, I sensed that no matter how much I had already uncovered, there was always more to be learned about this disease and about life. I decided to stay in therapy until I was done, hopefully before retirement.

However, as slowly as I was progressing, I seriously considered taking out a second mortgage to pay for all that fabulous enlightenment.

During one session, she looked at me as if she were looking into my soul and asked, "Why do you believe you needed this disease to cope with your life?"

She had gotten too close to the truth, and I reacted immediately. "Hang on. Are you telling me you think I brought this on myself as a way of ducking out of my life?"

She smiled. "I didn't say that. You did. But it's a good start. Maybe you were so exhausted and so disappointed with your life that you decided to check out of it altogether and hide in bed. Or it could be something else. Some believe that we come up with a plan for our life before we enter this world. The theory is that life is like a classroom, and we use situations to teach us what we need to learn. Could it be possible that you are trying to learn something big, so you set yourself up to experience a serious illness to help you find it? Of course, the answer could include all of the above or none of it. Life isn't linear; it's a hologram. There are usually many factors involved in why things happen."

I heard her words as they bounced through my head, but I had a hard time comprehending them. Just then, my phone rang. Pulling it out of my bag, I debated what to do.

She looked at me calmly and asked, "You gonna answer that?"

"It's my husband. He never calls. Hang on."

I turned toward the wall as if that would make taking a call in the middle of a session less noticeable. "What's up, honey? I'm pretty busy right now."

I could tell he was at the office by his tone of voice. "Sorry to interrupt, but I am in a meeting that will run longer than I had planned. Can you find someone else to pick up the girls from softball practice today?"

Mild panic set in. "That's like in an hour, and I won't be able to get there in time. Can't you call your mom?"

"No. She is out of town. Can you call yours?"

"I'll see what I can do, but can you give me more notice next time?"

"Sure, hon. I will be happy to anticipate that a meeting might run long and give you a heads-up several days in advance."

"Thanks for the sarcasm, dear. Talk to you later."

I didn't look at Mona right away. When I did, she was smiling.

"All good?"

"All good. I just need to make a quick call to my mother. It really does take a village."

After successfully rerouting my family, I tried to get back to business and remember everything she had said before we were interrupted. "I can't imagine I would ever consider this thing a great idea, no matter how much I thought I might learn from it. But I suppose it's possible."

She continued her train of thought. "When we are born, we are the opposite of our spirit's true nature. Sometimes we have to experience who we aren't in order to learn who we are. For example, you had to become weak so you could find your strength. When you view your struggles, look to the opposite of what those struggles entail. It is then that you will understand your essence and realize who your spirit truly is. This will lead you to your purpose.

Of course, you can have more than one purpose, too. Monaism!"

Easy for her to say. I was the one who had to figure out how that applied to my life.

After our session ended, I drove for a while, eventually finding myself at the beach. Something about the salt air and the sound of waves crashing always helped when my head was spinning.

How did all this happen? One day I was at Trader Joes getting bread and peanut butter for sandwiches, and the next I was on some spiritual journey with a nutty yet incredibly deep therapist, questioning my very existence.

My biggest concern used to be how I would duck out of chairing a committee at the kids' school. Now I comprehended concepts I didn't even know existed a few months ago.

Or at least I was trying to.

As I sat in the sand, I contemplated the grains running between my toes and wondered how many others before me had done the same while considering their own lives. Our time on this planet is more expansive than I'd realized. We get so caught up in the day-to-day that we're blind to how much more there can be when we are willing to break free of our cocoons and stretch beyond our comfort zones. I didn't enjoy where I was physically, because I still felt crappy. But emotionally and spiritually, I was connecting on a level that most people will never experience. It felt as if electricity ran through my veins.

It's said there is a light and a shadow side to every situation. The intensity I felt from both made me burn with a desire to continue until I unearthed some type of resolve. As painful as the dark was, when I walked through each horrific experience from my past, I realized it carried a lesson for me. And every lesson made me stronger and more determined to take each step with grace and an open mind.

CHAPTER 20

AS THE WEEKS TURNED into months, Mona and I became fast friends. I grew to love our talks and looked forward to the time we spent together, calling them "Thursdays with Mona." She opened my mind to fresh ideas and possibilities about myself and my life. I expected the process to be overwhelming, but it wasn't as difficult as I had played it up to be in my mind. She had a way of making really hard concepts easy and sensible. I liked easy and sensible, because I had no time or energy for complicated and confusing. She separated parts of my life into categories so they would be easy to access, calling them "the realms." They were how we started many of our sessions together.

On the Thursday before Easter, I walked into her office and tripped over a huge stuffed bunny. Mona greeted me with a big smile and a warm hug. I wondered if the twinkle in her eye was just for me or if she gave everyone the same loving welcome.

"Hi, honey!" she said. "How art thou today?"

I played along. "Thouest art grand."

I was never very good with Medieval lingo, but I thought I would give it a try.

Her penetrating gaze made me pause. It was weird, as if my eyes held the key for her to unlock all the information in my mind. Or was it my soul? Maybe she could see both. Either way, there was no fooling that woman.

Casually, she asked, "Whatcha thinking about, honey?"

I sat cautiously, trying to avoid the pain in my left hip. "I had another bone marrow biopsy on Monday. It's hard to believe I had to put the autoimmune disease on hold this week because my oncologist was worried my cancer had returned. I'm having trouble wrapping my head around this one. Haven't I had enough? Do you really believe what happens in our lives adds up in our bodies when we don't release it in time? Do you honestly believe I did this to myself?"

"Did what?"

"Made myself sick because of all the unresolved issues I didn't work through earlier in my life. This is so unfair. Why me? I'm a good person; I don't deserve this."

"Oops." She plopped down on her furry tiger-print couch.

"Oops? Why oops?" I switched to the boring brown chair. It kind of summed us up.

"Sounds like someone is moving into a victim state. That's no fun."

"What part of this illness thing is fun? You have no idea how painful all of this is." Sometimes I found her cheery attitude annoying.

"Trust me when I say I understand how physically painful it can be. I had to learn how to walk again, too, remember? But it is important to avoid making it any heavier than it needs to be. You have to accept where you are and let it flow through you. But let's return to your original question. When we blame others for their influence on our lives, we become victims to them and lose our power and sense of self. If we become self-responsible for our actions, an inner strength develops. I have a feeling that when your inner strength grows, so will your outer strength."

"Are you planning to give me the flu theory again?"

"Great idea! Let's do it. Ready?"

I tried not to roll my eyes. "Ready."

"If someone sneezes on you and gives you the flu, do you blame that person and lie on the floor whining about how they hurt you, or do you take care of yourself and get better?"

"Maybe a little of both." I spoke only truth with her. Sometimes I whined, too.

"That's fine with me, but it will take longer that way. Kind of drafty on the floor, too, isn't it? Remember, other people can be conduits for you, but only you can change you. Isn't that our ultimate goal: changing us, not others? What happens in life can be horrific, but it happens just the same. It's up to us to figure out what to do with it afterward. We can't go backward and change it; we can only change us . . . hopefully for the better."

"I understand what you are saying, but can't I have a minute to be sad or upset about some of the tragic things happening these days?"

She jumped up and grabbed a tennis racquet.

"Uh, Mona, what are you planning to do with that racquet?" I was getting a bit nervous. I never knew quite what to expect.

She looked puzzled. "You are filled with emotions that swirl around your mind, which can cloud your present view of life. I'm teaching you how to rinse those impressions out of your head so you can think properly, silly. It is kind of like rinsing the dirty water out of the tub in the washing machine. How can you possibly get your clothes clean when you have polluted water mucking them up?"

"And I can do this by playing a game of tennis?"

She laughed. "Don't be ridiculous."

"*You* are holding a tennis racquet, and *I'm* ridiculous?"

She ignored my comment. "Sometimes, you have to go beyond what you know."

"Is that a Monaism?"

"Sort of. What I mean is that you don't know what you don't know. You have to go beyond what you know to push yourself out of your comfort zone and move past whatever is keeping you stuck."

"And I do that with a tennis racquet?"

"Exactly."

I did roll my eyes that time but gave in to her tactics. "Okay, let's hear it."

She jumped on top of the coffee table with the racquet in one hand, her arms flailing about.

"We all experience things in life that are upsetting, but it's likely we have already experienced something similar on some level in our past if those things are still bothering us. It's kind of like traveling around and around in a circle until you find a way out."

"I don't think I'm following. Can you paint me a picture of what you mean?" Sometimes I felt that we were reading the same page in different books.

"Let's say you are married and your husband leaves you. It is terrible, and you are devastated, but it also reminds you of the time your father left when you were a child or when your dog died. Your husband is now the trigger for similar experiences in the past that you never dealt with. It has a domino effect in which one situation triggers a bunch of others with the same issue attached to it. They all come flooding back at the same time. If you don't process the base issue, which, for this illustration, happens to be abandonment, it may repeat in some fashion until you do. You will keep moving around the circle until you find your way out."

"So three different kinds of cancer and two autoimmune diseases means I must be really dense, because I keep rotating around the health circle with no knowledge of why or how to escape?"

She laughed. "Well! Who's the judgy judger now? There can't be judgment involved in processing your lessons or emotions. Once you judge, it is all over. You will make yourself crazy, literally. Over time, suppressed thoughts, feelings, and memories can affect your overall body chemistry. Another example would be physically moving slower because you feel weighed down by life and the pressure you feel from it. Or you can go the other way and become hyper and flighty while you try to avoid those emotions. A feeling of mental heaviness or stress can chemically affect your metabolism and cause weight gain and other real physical issues, as well. The goal is to rinse those sentiments out of your body and move on."

"You want me to rinse out the diseases I'm dealing with? Where would I even start, and how could anyone find the lesson here?"

She jumped off the table and grabbed a big pillow. "This is for you to process through, my dear. We can't really discover the answer to your question until you sort through all of your thoughts and beliefs and take a look at them.

"And I do that with a racquet and a pillow?"

"Yep. That is the first part, anyway. Rinsing is one of the most essential elements of processing. To truly understand ourselves and our histories, traumas, and victories, we have to go beyond our intellect. Sure, we're aware of what happened to us, but to release it, we need to go to the sensory level, as well. Human beings are part spirit and part animal. We need to let our emotions out on a purely animal level to see them for what they are, without logic, fear, or judgment. The more comfortable we are doing this, the more we can understand ourselves and others."

"My past is in the past. Why would I want to drag all that up again? It will just upset me more, and there is nothing I can do about it anyway."

Mona sat next to me and held my hand. It was as if she could feel my pain from all the memories I had stuffed way back in my psyche. "Oh, honey, repressed feelings don't go away, especially if you push them down. They just grow bigger until they explode or you implode."

"Implode?"

"Yes. Your body can collapse under the stress of all the built-up energetic sludge, kind of like a volcano exploding from the pressure. The lava from the eruption flows free, destroying everything in its path."

I was still back at energetic sludge. It was a fairly accurate term for the pent-up issues I'd never dealt with.

A light bulb went off over my head. "I understand what you are saying. I'm just not sure what to do with it."

"Well, the goal here is to release thoughts and attitudes from your body in a constructive way that doesn't hurt you or anyone else; remember, we never pass on our abuse."

"Killjoy. Okay, I'm still listening. Although sometimes it is kind of fun to pass on a little abuse."

She handed me the racquet, the pillow, and a piece of paper. "Enough talking; time to move."

"Where are we going?"

"Not we. You. You are taking a trip into your subconscious to pull out the demons so you can see them."

"Why would I want to do that? It sounds really scary."

"I know it does. But the scary monsters have been there the whole time. Isn't it better to face them and move them out of your body instead of letting them hide in the shadows of your mind?"

I curled into a fetal position in my chair. My voice became barely more than a whisper. "But what if I can't handle them? What if I freak out?"

She squeezed my hand and spoke more softly. "That's why this is very controlled. We create a safe place for you to take a look at what is in there and move it out. It's a process where we can start small and go deeper over time. And don't worry; I've got you. I understand exactly where you are right now and what we need to do. Are you ready, honey?"

"Do I have a choice?"

"We all have choices. We can choose to remain victims or possibly become abusers ourselves, or we can learn how to process through our emotions and achieve wisdom. It's up to you."

"Since you put it that way, what exactly would you like me to do?"

"First, you have to fill out the rinse paper I gave you. It will tap into the psyche and tell you what your real issues are and where you need to go with them."

I looked at the paper. It was a fill-in-the-blank exercise that seemed simple enough. The only problem was that I couldn't answer the first question.

"It says to finish a sentence that starts with 'I am angry because.'" I'm not angry. Can I skip that one?"

"We are all angry, scared, hurt, and embarrassed about something on some level. It's in there; to dig it up, all you have to do is write it out. It can be anything. If rude people make you mad, start with that. Or you can go back to your past . . . maybe something your father did when you were young or a friend who upset you a long time ago. The point is to start bringing up hidden anger wherever you find it at that moment. The bigger stuff is usually right underneath. As I said before, if we leave all that negative energy alone, it will get stuck in the body and start to affect our decisions and health. If we pull it out and take a look, the negative stuff will teach us what we are here to learn, and we will grow from it. Eventually, the lessons turn into wisdom. Try it again. I'll bet you find something."

"Okay. Here goes. I'm angry because people step on my ability to speak up. No. *My father* never let me speak up."

"Good. Keep filling in the rest of the page. Don't do it out loud, though. When we write it out, we bypass the part of our brain that judges. That way, we'll *feel* the answers instead of thinking about them."

I wasn't feeling them, but I began to write.

And it made me feel . . . *bullied.*

You ruined my life because . . . *I lost the ability to have a voice in the world.*

I hate you because . . . *I feel insignificant now.*

I hate me because . . . *I let it happen.*

I am scared because . . . *I realize all of my health issues started in my throat. And I have allowed others to step on my voice, too.*

Which makes me think . . . *I somehow created these diseases to bring attention to my throat and voice or lack of them.*

I am scared because . . . *I am not sure I can fix this. And I don't want to recreate this pattern with my children.*

I am afraid of . . . *not being strong enough to speak up or survive this disease.*

I put the pen down and started to cry. I cried so hard I couldn't finish the rest of the page; I couldn't see it through my tears.

Mona handed me a tissue and the racquet. "Looks like someone is ready for part two. You are doing great, honey. You may not be aware of where you are right now in this process, but, as I told you before, I am. Trust me."

I tried to wipe the tears from my face. "What now?"

"First we gotta find a place where you'll feel safe to complete the rest of the process. I like to do it where nobody will be able to hear me . . . someplace small like a closet or my bedroom, so I'll feel safe. Close the door and lock it, so there are no interruptions. Right now, we can do it on the floor of my office, since everyone is gone for the day. Put the paper on the floor next to the pillow and get on your knees in front of it. Grab the racquet and just start whacking away."

I looked at the pillow. "This is silly. I'll feel ridiculous doing that. Do you have any other options?"

"Nope. Just try it a couple of times for fun. You will be surprised how easy it becomes. Raise the racquet over your head and hit the pillow as hard as you can. Go!"

I felt as awkward as I'd expected, but I figured I didn't have much to lose. I sat on the floor and hit it softly.

"Is that all you got? Wimp."

"Seriously? You are goading me?" I hit it harder.

"Keep trying. That was better but not much."

Now *she* was the one I was going to have anger towards. I hit the pillow harder. Then even harder. Adrenalin coursed through my veins.

"Now start reading from the paper while you hit the pillow. Talk, whack, talk, whack."

As I started to read, the anger welled up in my throat. It made me want to hit harder. The harder I hit, the louder my voice became.

The louder my voice, the more I wanted to kill that pillow, unleashing a cyclone of rage that had been living in my mind and destroying anything in its path for far too long.

Then I suddenly stopped. She came over to me, trying to assess what was wrong.

"You okay, honey?"

I lunged for my purse, accidently knocking it off the chair and spilling the contents. "Oh, my God! Clearing all the crap from my head made me remember something." I grabbed my phone from the floor.

Her look of concern was unmistakable. "A childhood trauma?"

Feverishly texting, I said, "No. I forgot to pick up the dog from the groomer. She hates it there, and when she gets mad at me, she poops all over the house for days. I'm texting my sister to see if she can get there before they close."

Mona sat on the floor with her legs crossed. "Well, that's a first. Maybe that is how dogs do anger rinsing. Can we get back to work now?"

After putting the contents of my purse back where they belonged, I continued where I'd left off. Imagining my biological dad's face on the pillow made me even angrier than before, and I wanted to hit even harder. I started yelling at him. For a minute, I forgot where I was. I returned to the time when I was small and he wouldn't let me speak up about his abuse and neglect. I was reliving the whole thing, but that time I got to fight back by saying my piece. My silent throat finally had a voice. It felt as if I was vomiting the memories onto the pillow and leaving them there.

Eventually, I stopped. I threw the racquet down and lay on the floor by the pillow. I was exhausted. Mona sat next to me and gently put her hand on my arm to bring me back to the present.

"You did awesome, honey. I am so proud of you." She was silent for a moment. "Isn't it interesting that all of your health issues stem from your throat? There must be a lot happening in that area energetically, which could be part of what is causing the physical issue. By having a voice this way, you can clean up that part. That is why we call it a rinse."

I was curled in fetal position but listening intently. My voice remained small, like a young girl's. "Is it possible this will cure me?"

Her next words emerged slowly. "It certainly won't hurt you to get that stuff out, but we may not see the fruits of our labors in this life. However, the lessons we learn we keep for all eternity. You are taking the necessary steps to control your own life; now you get to define how you want to be in this world, no matter what struggles you face. That is all we can ask for. Find your struggle, learn your lesson, and then discover your purpose."

I got off the floor and did a mental check-in. I felt really good, cleaned out, like you do after a case of the stomach flu. You're sure you will never stop throwing up, and then when you do, you feel completely purged. And a few pounds lighter. I walked out of her office that day looking like I had just been mugged and feeling on top of the world.

The experience inspired me to clean out my closet so I could make room for my new friends, the pillow and the racquet.

That night I decided to try it on my own. For some reason, I found myself stalling. It reminded me of my school days. I often avoided homework by doing anything else I could dream up instead. Once the laundry was done, the house cleaned, the kids in bed, and the dishes washed, I realized I had run out of excuses.

I placed an old seat cushion on the floor and sat quietly, taking ten deep breaths. Mona had explained that deep breathing slows the nervous system. I had made several copies of the rinse paper, and I took one out of my new rinse notebook. Answering each question as well as I could, I noticed I was delving deeper into the issue while working through the list. It was that onion peeling again. After I finished writing, I took a few practice swings to become comfortable with the sound and the sense of it in my body. I even wore leather gardening gloves to save my hands from blisters, as Mona had suggested. They had sayings on the front, like "The more one sows, the greater the harvest." True on many levels.

Eventually, I started hitting the pillow while reading the items on the paper out loud. I began to feel something release in my body. I wasn't sure what that meant but decided to continue without judgment or shame, which was not a natural response for me. I had to keep reminding myself my environment was safe and that even if I got lost for a minute, the present was always right there. And no one was listening.

Once my psyche was clean, my body relaxed. I hadn't worried about the time or the noise. I'd given myself the space and permission to release all the fear and anger I had held onto for so long.

After seeing all that was inside me, I became convinced that unresolved anger could be the downfall of civilization. How many wars have been started because someone was mad about something that happened years ago?

Later that night, I watched the news while lying in bed. Something tragic had happened in the Middle East, and there were scenes of women wailing in the streets, their bodies writhing on the ground in emotional anguish.

I wondered why our society is so uncomfortable showing emotion when other cultures do it regularly. *What are we afraid of? Do we view it as a sign of weakness?*

Perhaps that is why I hid in my closet while I rinsed away all the feelings I'd stuffed for so many years. It reminded me of the other cultures that hide their emotions in one way or another, too.

My mind went back to the time our Italian neighbors invited us to spend Thanksgiving with them. I watched as they screamed and yelled and cried and laughed with each other, all before the pie was served. Back then, I felt intimidated by their behavior. Now, I understand that they were simply letting their emotions flow with no judgment.

I could learn from them; they will probably live a whole lot longer than I will. And be happier in the long run because of the way they process their emotions.

CHAPTER 21

Don't let what you can't do stop you from what you can do.
John Wooden

AFTER WEEKS OF RINSING success, I couldn't wait for my next session with Mona. The processing of old emotions was painful at times, but I pushed through and followed her program on a daily basis, creating a positive shift in my body. Maybe my mind had shifted, too. I hoped so. Something had definitely changed, and I felt stronger mentally and physically. Best of all, I needed to take less medicine to make it through each day, which I found very interesting.

Overjoyed by my progress, I almost exploded into her office when I arrived, pushing the door into a life-sized Uncle Sam standee. Mona sat behind her desk playing with the American flags she'd used to decorate her red, white, and blue foil tree. I didn't ask.

She looked up, startled. "Well, hello there, my little ray of sunshine! Someone looks much brighter and clearer today."

I tripped over my words to get them all out. "Oh, my God! You have no idea how much anger I have built up over the years! Well, maybe you do, but I had no idea how truly pissed off I've been! There are blisters on my blisters from hitting that stupid pillow. My family thought I'd gone crazy at first. But then they noticed my more relaxed mood after each session in my closet. Now they encourage me to keep going. Yesterday I got a little grumpy, and my son actually said I should go upstairs and do whatever I do in there to make me happy again."

She laughed. "How about that. The child is sending his mother to her room for a time out. Sounds like a pretty smart kid to me.

Feeling very evolved in that moment, I sauntered over to the leopard-skin couch instead of the plain one and sat down. I'd finally made some progress as I traveled an uncharted road and learned the lessons Mona had taught me, moving on to the next level. It reminded me of playing Pac-Man as a kid, eating all the little cherries to reach the levels with more important fruit.

As Mona watched me, I imagined she read my mind by looking at the smug expression on my face. I suspected she was about to deflate my puffed-out chest and bring me back to earth.

She began with, "So, where are we on the realms today?"

The reentry had happened faster than expected. "The what?"

"The realms. Remember me telling you about the different aspects of your being and how they relate to each other and the world?"

I crossed my arms as if pouting. "Can't we go back to the rinsing thing? I have that one nailed."

"Which is exactly why we are charging forward."

So much for my ego. "I remember them."

"And why are they important?"

I had to make up an answer for that question. "Because it is a way to break apart our emotions. It sort of unravels the twists we do in our heads and puts our emotions in categories to help us take a look at them. This helps balance and reprioritize our thinking."

"Exactly. I find it is the best way to check in. Our goal is to try to stay in balance for at least a few minutes a day. It's also a great way to assess where we hold our priorities and how we make our life choices. Memorizing them in order helps us remember the proper sequence for our life. Can you name them?"

I did a mental checklist to see if I had them all before replying. "Okay. The realms, in order, are:

Spiritual, defined by you as truth and love. It's the most important from your perspective.

Mental, our logical and rational thought, the second most important.

Emotional, which includes our feelings, whether past, present, or future.

Physical, our body and animal energy.

Sexual, meaning how we relate to both gender and sexuality.

Financial, which can include money but also our powerful-versus-powerless struggles."

"Yes, my little gifted one. And which one is running your life right now?"

"I would say emotional is probably at the head of the pack currently, or I wouldn't be wondering if I'm losing my mind all the time."

"So true. When we lead with our emotional realm, we can feel a little crazy. Then our mental realm will jump in and confirm it, because it is judging the hell out of us. Let's say, for example, that we had the thought that we made ourselves physically sick due to the situations that have happened to us in the past. If our emotional realm were in first place, we would start reliving the past circumstances that we believed made us ill and get lost in them. This would stop us from growing, because we are now caught up in the trance of a particular moment that affected us, with no awareness of the spinning in our minds. Then our mental state would come in and start calling us nuts. After all, it wouldn't make sense that we were stuck, so our mind would try to come up with a logical reason to explain the way we are feeling, which would be impossible to do, because it isn't logical. This process would take a lot of energy, which would drain the physical body if it went on for too long. Without any energy, the sexual realm wouldn't have a prayer either because we then pity ourselves and what has happened, which would make us dead inside and turn us into powerless, pitiful victims."

I took a deep breath. "Bingo! I'm exhausted after listening to you explain what goes on in my head without my knowledge."

I wondered if my ignorance was bliss or an internal nightmare I lived with daily. I did love it when she decoded my issues, though. More accurately, I both loved and hated it when that happened.

"But you forgot about the spiritual realm."

"That's because it is nowhere in sight. You would be surprised how many people don't even know they have a spiritual realm, so how could they possibly exercise it? Just so you are clear as to what I mean, want to play a game?"

"Sure!" I liked the game-playing part of our program. She described it a passive way to learn potentially confusing ideas by going through the back door of our brains. It made the learning part more fun.

"Think of a person, such as a celebrity, who is out of balance in his or her realms. We are all out of kilter at some point in our lives, but see if you can find an exaggerated version of it in someone else's personality so you can more easily see the realms at work in yourself. I'll give you the first one. When I think of someone who has the financial realm at the top of his list, I think of Donald Trump. I'll bet one of the reasons he is so powerful in the financial realm is because he feels powerless in another realm and is overcompensating. Get it?"

I pondered some options. "Okay. Someone with his sexual realm on top would be . . . Hugh Hefner?"

"Oh, that's a good one! What about mental?"

"Mental. Who is logical about everything? Does Spock on Star Trek count?"

"That works. He believes logic is the most important aspect of life. That belief would throw him out of balance in the emotional realm, which is why he didn't experience any feelings."

"Physical would be someone like Arnold Schwarzenegger when he was Mr. Olympian and starred in all those violent movies."

"Yes! And, for the bonus question, can you think of someone with their spiritual realm out of whack?"

"I thought spiritual belonged on top of the pyramid."

"It does. However, if it is the only thing you care about and you ignore the rest of them, you are still out of balance. You can't skip steps."

"Okay. How about the Pope?"

"No, he still has a pretty good business sense. Try again."

"How about the cult leader who made everyone drink the Kool-Aid so they could all leave the planet together and get into heaven via a spaceship or something. Do you remember that?"

"Yeah, that's what we call a total tragedy on all levels. Not very spiritual in my book. Keep going."

I was running out of ideas. "A monk who takes a vow to leave everything and everyone behind to live in a cave somewhere so he can meditate all day long?"

"That one is pretty good. That person isn't really living a full and complete life, is he?"

"Not much. So if I were to put my realms in order right now, they would be:

1. Emotional, because I'm thinking with my emotions first right now.
2. Mental, because I'm overthinking everything.
3. Physical, because I am always aware of my body and what I can do physically within the limits of my disease.
4. Spiritual, because I really want to figure this thing out and follow whatever my truth is.
5. Financial, because I am very aware of how much my medical bills are costing.
6. Sexual, because with all that is on my plate the thought of sexuality doesn't even hit my radar.

"Very good. As you can see, if the order is off, so are you. That's why it's important to take stock of yourself at some point each day. Regular check-ins allow us the space to rearrange some thoughts and put them back in order if your realms are off. Can you do that for me this week, baby?"

"I will try."

I really did want to try. They say it takes twenty-one days to create or break a habit. I truly wanted reordering my realms to become a new habit.

"I'll expect a full report next week. Never forget, you're a rock star!"

Rock star status was never something I thought possible, but the convincing way Mona said it made me believe it could happen one day. I was so grateful to be learning what she knew and secretly wished everybody had a Mona in their lives so we could all grow together.

Why don't we have someone teaching us all this stuff? Why do we have to wait until we are messed up to figure it out? Most parents can't be responsible for passing on this kind of knowledge, because we haven't learned it either. Imagine what the world would be like if we figured it out in elementary school. We could become mature adults who make good choices.

The human race has made amazing progress in technology, medicine, and science. Yet when it comes to emotional intelligence, we are barely half a step up from the Neanderthal age. I may not be able to change the world (not that the world would want me to change it anyway), but Mona had changed me and many others.

Perhaps one day we can pass her wisdom on to our families, and they can pass it on to theirs, and together we can make this place a little more livable.

CHAPTER 22

No one can go back and make a brand new start.
Anyone can start from now and make a brand new ending.
Unknown

MY GOAL FOR THE NEXT couple of months was to stay out of the hospital. Naively, I thought that working through my emotional triggers would cure my physical issues. If what Mona said was true and emotional stress changes our biochemistry in a negative way, then why couldn't releasing that stress change it back? Maybe it can to a degree, but given all my medical problems, I would probably need full-time therapy for the next two hundred years to make a dent in my health.

One thing was certain. I'd fallen short of my "just say no to hospitals" goal again.

Unfortunately, when the paramedics picked me up, they took me to my least favorite hospital . . . not that I enjoyed any of them. Hoping not to stay as long as I had before, I decided to accept my fate and give the place another chance. I didn't really have a choice anyway; I wasn't breathing well enough on my own to put up much of a fuss.

I had become the secret shopper of hospitals, landing in six different facilities during the previous year or so. That particular institution had not earned high marks, at least not from me. On my first visit to their Emergency Room, I was unconscious when the ambulance delivered me to the door. My husband told them I had myasthenia gravis and said there were many drugs I couldn't take due to my condition. They gave them to me anyway.

With the power of the Internet at their disposal, I'd assumed that when a patient entered the emergency room with a rare autoimmune disease, the doctors would look it up if they weren't familiar with it. They could at least have read the warnings on the card I carry with me at all times explaining what not to do during a crisis.

They did neither.

When my blood pressure dropped to 60/40 and I was at risk for a heart attack or stroke, they realized they should investigate and learn if there was a better way to treat me. I lived, but just barely, and vowed never to darken their doorway again.

Mona said we are forced to face our deepest fears in order to overcome them. Maybe that was why I entered the same emergency room again. The second time, however, I was conscious. After filling out the necessary paperwork, a nurse escorted me to a room in the back. The doctor on staff was carrying my encyclopedia-sized file when he walked in. He gazed at me over the top of his glasses.

"What seems to be the matter with you today? You look pretty healthy to me!"

Why is it that healthy-looking people are instantly dismissed by the medical community? Aren't most health issues on the inside of the body?

Trying to be as polite as possible, I said, "Thank you. I'm glad I look well. Unfortunately, I am having trouble breathing."

"Why?"

"Why what?"

"Why can't you breathe?"

"Why can't I breathe right now or why do I have trouble breathing in general?" I wasn't sure which one of us was making the situation more complicated than it needed to be.

"Both."

"Well, I can't breathe in general because I have myasthenia gravis. I can't breathe today because my insurance company recently canceled the IV medicine I've been getting every two weeks. Without that medicine, my muscles are very weak, which is making it harder and harder for me to function. My strength lessens every day, along with my ability to take in a breath. I got worried because my lips and fingers were turning blue, and I can only talk in the morning for a few hours before I start to run out of enough air to speak."

"Why did your insurance company do that?"

It was an obvious question. The bigger question is *Why do insurance companies do most of the things they do to their clients?*

"They said it was because they reclassified my medicine as experimental, which is their way of saying they no longer want to pay for it."

"Is it experimental?"

"No, it is the standard in the industry for what I have, but it costs about $5,000 a month, and I have been on it for a while now."

Compassion filled his eyes, and he sat down next to me. "The same thing happened to my mother a few years ago. Her chemo drugs were costing the insurance company a fortune, and she was old. They reclassified those, as well. We tried to fight them, but it took time to go through the 'proper' channels. She never saw the day the State Department of Insurance overturned their decision to discontinue treatment. She'd passed away a few days before."

I could feel his pain. "I'm sorry. I have three kids of my own, and I'm trying to be as strong for them as your mom probably was for you. It's really hard sometimes. Especially when it feels like a company's profit is more important than my life and my family."

He looked off into the distance. I wondered what he was thinking. Suddenly his eyes became very clear. "You know, when I got into this doctor business, I took an oath that the health of my patients would be my number one consideration and I would do no harm. I just wish everyone else invested in making medical decisions for my patients had taken the same oath." He closed my file. "We will do our best here to help you breathe a little better so you can get back to your children."

I put my hand on his arm as if to somehow convey my appreciation. He smiled sweetly and disappeared behind the curtain. I heard him rattling off orders to the nurses to expedite the process of moving me to another floor. I was very grateful but secretly hoped I wouldn't be sent to the Intensive Care Unit, even though I knew that was going to be the case.

CHAPTER 23

TWO HOURS LATER, I was admitted to the Intensive Care Unit.

Although I never like to look a gift horse in the mouth and was truly grateful to be receiving the much-needed medicine, I didn't want to be back in the ICU. There are many reasons it wasn't my favorite place:

1. The staff drew labs at 4:30 every morning. It's a terrible way to wake up. . . if I was lucky enough to fall asleep at all.
2. The life support machines on the floor are deafening.
3. The sound of lungs being suctioned 24/7 makes it very hard to eat.
4. I didn't want to eat anyway, because the food they served was "mechanical soft," which means they toss regular meals in a blender, pour it on a plate, and serve it to you. It's beyond gross.
5. At that particular hospital, there are no private rooms on the ICU floor, since most of the patients are unconscious. My "room" was a six-by-ten-foot space encircled by curtains. There was little air to breathe, even if breathing weren't so difficult for me.

If that weren't enough to make my stay miserable, the ICU nurse assigned to me was a tall, gangly man in starched scrubs and bright blue Crocs, who had a passion for following the rules. He greeted me with a thermometer and a blood pressure cuff.

"Hi, Mary. I will be your nurse for the remainder of my twelve-hour shift today and for the rest of the week."

I tried to be cheerful, but I had a bad feeling about him.

"My name is Lisa."

"Your wrist tag says Mary; is that not you?"

"Mary is my first name, but I go by Lisa. They put Mary on there because that is what it says on my driver's license."

"Well, if that is what it says, then that is what I am going to call you. We have to keep it legal."

"But no one knows me as Mary, including my doctors." I felt tired and my patience was waning.

"Then you should have thought of that before you put it on your driver's license. By the way, my name is Richard, but you can call me Dick."

Somehow I didn't think calling him *Dick* was going to be a problem, even if it wasn't printed on his driver's license.

"I need to go to the bathroom, Dick. Can I do that before you hook me up to all those lines?" It had been more than a few hours since I was able to go, and I really needed to pee.

"Nope, afraid not. You are going to have to use a bedpan. I will get it when I'm done."

"I would hate for you to have to clean up a bedpan, and the bathroom is less than twenty feet away. I'll be right back." I started to wiggle around like a child waiting for the teacher to hand over the big yellow hall pass.

He placed a strong hand on my shoulder to keep me from getting up. "Let's get one thing clear, dear, so we can keep your stay peaceful. This is not a hotel. You do not call the shots. We do not let you do things the doctor did not put in your orders, and you will use a bedpan whether you like it or not."

I instantly knew why they had assigned Dick to the floor with mostly unconscious, intubated patients. He completely lacked social skills.

I thought it over for a minute, trying to decide how best to handle the situation. There are many ways to have a voice. I could be angry, act like a victim, or go for a passive/aggressive stance. In the end, I decided to do something different and try the straightforward approach.

"Well, Dick, I could wait until you're done with whatever it is you plan to do. However, with my particular disease, my bladder isn't very patient. We could instead go with the other option, which might be better and cleaner for both of us. All I need to do is walk a few steps to the bathroom right over there and be done in about three minutes."

He waved me off. "You see, this is why I like the geriatric patients. They don't put up such a fuss about things. I'll get your bedpan, and we can hook you up afterward. Hope you can handle it yourself, though. I don't do lady parts. How's that for a compromise?"

There didn't appear to be much compromise in his plan, but if I didn't do something soon, we'd both be dealing with a mess. Reluctantly, I agreed.

He seemed pleased with himself after he'd gotten me settled in. "There now, that's better. Is there anything else you need?"

"I haven't had anything to eat or drink all day. Do you think I could get a little food and some water?"

"No water. Not on your orders."

"No water . . . ever? Then what can I drink?"

"You are on a mechanical soft diet. That means you get thickened water if you want it with your meals."

"Thickened water? Isn't that ice?" I'd taken physics in high school, but I had a feeling the hospital had something else in mind.

"Thickened water includes cornstarch and sugar. It doesn't taste that bad once you get used to it. I'll bring you some with your pureed turkey sandwich at dinner."

I couldn't believe it. They were adding cornstarch and sugar to water and serving it to sick people who are trying to get better? I'd read studies showing that sugar destroys the germ-killing ability of white blood cells for up to five hours after ingestion. For someone with immune issues, that didn't seem like a good idea. In addition, cornstarch mixed with water can cause severe constipation. Mine was already severe enough.

Why wouldn't a hospital give patients nutritious food if improving their health is the primary goal? No wonder our health care system is a total disaster.

I was too tired to argue and decided to text my husband and ask him to smuggle a bottle of water and a Jamba Juice smoothie to my room. "Can you hand me my purse, please?"

He whirled around and grabbed it. "I was about to get to that. We have to catalogue everything you brought in." He dumped the contents on the bed next to me and started rifling through them.

Horrified, I stammered, "Wha—what are you doing?"

"I'm making a note of everything you have in your purse. I see you have an iPad, too. You can't use that here . . . or the cell phone."

"Why? My iPad doesn't have Internet, and I can only text on my phone."

"I will have to have someone come by to check them out. Any electronics have to be cleared before you can use them in the ICU. It will take some time."

He frowned when he heard what must have been an unfamiliar tune. I knew exactly what it was.

He asked, "Do you hear that?"

I did, but I wasn't sure I wanted to fess up. "Hear what?"

"That music. What is that?"

Nonchalantly, I said, "I think it is Bob Marley."

"Who?"

I wasn't surprised that he hadn't recognized the tune or its performer. "The song is called 'Don't Worry About a Thing.' Bob Marley sings it. It's the ringtone on my phone."

"Don't answer that, young lady!"

As appreciative as I was that he'd called me a young lady, there was no way I was not going to answer my phone. My son was calling me. Even if I have to beg for breath, I will always answer the phone when my children call. Always.

"It will just take a sec, Dick. My kids don't know I am here, and they are probably starting to panic. I left them a note, but they came home from school to an empty house. I need to tell him not to worry."

"No, you don't. There are no phone conversations in the ICU." He tried unsuccessfully to grab the phone out of my hands.

As I pulled back, I hid the phone under my covers. "Look, this will only take a second. I am not letting my children think something terrible is happening to their mother."

Even if something was.

"Look, lady . . ."

Holding my hand in front of his face to put him on pause, I answered the cell phone with the other. "Hi, honey. I'm sorry I wasn't there when you guys got home. Please don't be worried. Your mom is going to be just fine."

There was a pause on the other end of the phone. Then my son responded. "What? Oh. Glad to hear it. But I need to ask you something really important."

I could tell that Dick's patience was about to run out. Pulling the phone away from my ear, I said, "Dick, my kids are really scared. Let me reassure them I am well, and I will be off in a minute."

Not giving him time to respond, I turned my attention back my son. "Tan, I am here for you. Ask away. What's up?"

"Mom, I can't find my sweatshirt. You know the quarter zip? I put it in the laundry room to be washed the other day. Did you clean it? I need it for tonight."

Turning my head away from Dick, I answered in a half whisper, "Bottom drawer."

"What?"

A little louder, I said, "I washed it and put it in the bottom drawer with your other sweaters. If you cleaned your room once in a while, you would know you actually have clothes that don't live on your floor."

Ignoring my last comment, my son continued. "One more thing. My coach said you and Dad need to finish your volunteer hours. Since you didn't make it to the last meeting, he signed you up for bathroom duty at my next race. Do you think you will be home in time?"

"I'm sure I will, honey. Tell your coach not to worry. Oh, and thanks for the concern."

Unfazed by my sarcasm, he replied, "You're welcome, Mom, and I'll just order a pizza, since you're not home to make dinner. Talk to you later. Love you!"

With that, my son was gone. Dick smiled, as if he felt somewhat vindicated.

"Still want to keep that phone?"

I did. As much as I dreaded the prospect of bathroom duty, I rather liked the fact that I didn't have to turn my back on my life completely to deal with my health. I was still a part of the family puzzle.

Then I turned my attention to the unconscious patients in nearby cubicles, their every breath commanded by machines. It felt surreal. One minute, I had been folding laundry and thinking about school plays and what to make for dinner that night. The next, I was once more in the ICU. I couldn't help wondering if my disease would turn even uglier, someday making their current reality my fate.

I had to get out of there.

I turned to Dick, who was busy recording various numbers on my monitors. "Is my doctor coming by soon?"

With his back to me, he responded flatly, "He will be here when he gets here."

"And my husband? I haven't seen him since I was in the ER."

"You are in the ICU. The people in here are very sick. We can't have him eavesdropping on everyone's condition, so he will have limited access to you."

I might have been under intensive care, but Nurse Dick seemed to think we were in the psychiatric ward.

"I assure you the only medical condition my husband is interested in is mine. This isn't my first time in the ICU, and he is always with me and very sensitive to the other patients' privacy. I will make you a deal and leave my iPad off, but if you take my phone so I can't talk to him, I will walk . . . or crawl . . . out of here right now, and my doctor will have you shot."

I was getting cranky, and I knew my neurologist would have my back on that one.

"Okay. Calm down, drama queen. I tell you what, let's finish this conversation after you take your medications." He handed me a fistful of pills I didn't recognize.

"What are these?"

"Blood thinner, stomach protonic, something to help you sleep, a pain killer, and your regular dose of Synthroid. You will get the Mestinon later."

I was confused. "I don't take blood thinners, protonics, or sleeping pills. I'm not in any pain currently and took my Synthroid this morning. I will, however, need the Mestinon as soon as it runs out in my system, which is about an hour from now."

He peered at me over his glasses. "Are you refusing medical treatment?"

I'd had enough of our pointless dialogue. "If not taking medicine that I normally don't take without talking to my doctor first and double dosing on a medication I've already taken today means I am refusing medical treatment, then, yes. I guess I am."

"Then I will have to call your doctor regarding this matter."

I had been working with my doctor for quite a while and had been in the hospital six times under his care. We understood and respected each other. "I think that is a great idea. Why don't you ask him about the water and electronics while you are at it?"

When you are in the bull pen, which is code for a big room with nothing but curtains to separate the patients, everyone can hear everything. That can be both good and bad. Although Dick had stepped away from my cubicle to call my doctor, he was well within earshot. The conversation with my neurologist went well . . . for me.

"Doctor, I have your patient Mary here, and she is refusing medical treatment . . . Mary. You admitted her a few hours ago."

I thought I would help him out. "He doesn't know me by that name, because it isn't what I go by. Remember?"

"Okay, Lisa is refusing medical treatment. She won't take some of her medications. Which ones? The protonic, blood thinner, pain medicine, and muscle relaxant."

"Well, sir, we give those prophylactically; it is the hospital policy. Everyone on this ward gets them. Yes, sir. I understand. Whatever you say, sir."

I couldn't see Dick's face, but I had a feeling he wasn't happy with the conversation.

A few minutes later, he stuck his head around the curtain. "He said you don't have to take the protocol that seems to work for everyone but you. You can also keep your phone."

"Thanks," I said as sweetly as I could manage.

I really was grateful to have my phone. It was the only connection I had to my family, and it can get very isolating and scary in the hospital. I immediately texted my husband to tell him I loved him and to ask him to bring me some water. It was going to be a long night.

After a day or so in the middle of the bull pen, I settled in, although I couldn't believe what was going on around me. I watched in shock from the corner of my curtain wall as my eightyish-year-old neighbor ingested a cocktail of Ambien, Benadryl, Oxycontin, and Norco, which is a combination of acetaminophen and hydrocodone. Her nurse rattled off the names of each pill in a sing-song manner to get her to swallow them "like a good girl." She could not have weighed more than eighty pounds, and she was given those drugs every four hours around the clock.

What are we doing to our aged friends who are too frail to have their own voices?

I worried that if I didn't get out of there soon, I would die from an overdose or some unexplainable cause. I could breathe easier now that the medication had kicked in, and the color was returning to my hands and face. I just didn't know if I could handle being there another minute.

The one thing I had going for me was the charge nurse. She and every other ICU nurse except mine seemed to like hanging out with me, which made the time go faster. I enjoyed laughing and cracking jokes with them.

Dick, on the other hand, never warmed up to me. "Time for our bedtime meds!" he would sing in delight as he whisked back my curtain every night. I think his favorite part of the day was when he got to drug me to sleep. Although I didn't take most of the hospital protocol meds, I did take something to drown out the noise and light that otherwise kept me awake all night.

Within minutes, I would slide into my beautiful dreamland, where all was well and I was healthy and free.

Even if it was narcotically induced.

CHAPTER 24

Living twice at once you learn; you're safe from pain in the dream domain
A soul set free to fly
Queensrÿche

WHEN I FIRST CROSSED OVER to the other side of my mind, I saw nothing but darkness and felt completely vulnerable in my dream state. Soon, I began watching myself in what seemed like a movie where I was dressed in business clothes and running down Pacific Coast Highway. Dropping fully into the scene, I found it was surprisingly easy to run in heels, and I felt overjoyed to be hitting the road again, even though I was still a little scared in the dark. Suddenly, I sensed someone running behind me. When he caught up, he performed cartwheels and backflips, seemingly filled with energy and as fast as the wind.

"Melville? What are you doing? What's with all the acrobatics?"

He never missed a beat or ran out of breath. "You tell me, Meliana. This is your show."

"Good point." It seemed I was in for another lesson. My dreams tend to be more instructional than entertaining. Why can't I just fly around and simply be entertained like everyone else?

He observed my clothing as he ran beside me. "Why are you all dressed up?"

"I'm going back to work. I am finally ready and have a lot of job interviews today. There are so many options, and I am very excited."

He smiled and slowed his pace. Then he sped up again, putting on another demonstration for me with his energetic flipping. I slowed to watch the miraculous man spinning in the air and wondered what prompted him to perform such feats.

"That's impressive. Why are you doing it?"

"The purpose of my show is to demonstrate how easy it is to redirect you from your mission."

"Come again?" I hated sounding so lost. I'd been a pretty good student in college, but interacting with Melville made me very humble about my ability to comprehend anything.

"You were so excited to be all dressed up and literally running toward a new career and a new life. A minute later, you slowed your pace to match mine and became distracted. Where's your focus?"

The symbolism could not have been more accurate.

"I understand perfectly. I was traveling a new path with a sense of direction. Then, just like that, I was thrown off course by a sideshow."

I wondered if sideshows throw everyone off track in life or if it's just me they derail. How does that keep happening?

My kids and their friends have an inside joke they came up with after watching a Disney movie called *Up*. In the movie, a dog named Doug gets easily distracted by squirrel sightings. When our family gets off topic now, someone yells, "Squirrel!" They think it is a hilarious buzzword that reminds us to get back on point.

Apparently, I encounter a lot of squirrels.

"So what you are saying is that my path is far from straight, because I seem to be easily lost in the woods, chasing squirrels?"

"You are not a dog, Meliana. You have the power to do whatever you choose, but you constantly lose yourself in others. All someone has to do is throw the ball, and you are off and running in another direction to catch it. Look how easily I changed your pace. You need to be more conscious of your actions, or you will miss what is happening in your own life."

And there it was. The reason I never get anywhere. I'm too busy chasing my tail.

Suddenly, it all made sense. We have to focus ourselves, not in a selfish way but in a way that assures our soul's survival. Finally, I could see my path clearly. What I was missing was the intention to stay on it.

As if I'd been speaking aloud, Melville agreed.

"You need to run your own race now, Meliana. Stay on your path, wherever it leads you, until the end. It is part of who you are. It's your soul's truth. No one can ever take it away from you but you. You are truly in charge of your own destiny no matter what your external circumstances might be. Never forget where you are headed, and you will eventually find your way there."

I often tell my children to run their own race, and Melville was politely shoving my own words in my face. Perhaps I needed to start looking in the mirror before expressing my Mommyisms.

Suddenly, the obnoxiously loud beeping of my monitors woke me up, returning me to reality. I wasn't home in my bed. I was still in the hospital. Looking around for something to write on, I found a copy of my daily blood work report. I retrieved a pencil from my "Welcome to our Hospital" pack and scribbled, "Run your own race no matter what hurdles you encounter. No more squirrels." Dick would probably request a psychiatric evaluation if he found my note, but I didn't care. The dream was too important to forget.

CHAPTER 25

THE NEXT DAY DICK decided to let me have a visitor. She breezed into the ward looking like part white angel and part cabaret dancer. Mona's energy and sparkle lit up the room. She even got a smile from Dick and her own chair to sit in.

"Good morning, sunshine! How are we feeling today?"

God bless the therapist who makes house calls. "I'm feeling better, thanks. At least I can breathe better. This place has been a little mentally challenging, though."

Boy, was that an understatement.

She smiled. "What? You don't like it here in Camelot? Your prince is here to honor your every wish. You're not okay with that?"

"Come again?" She had me a little confused, as usual.

"If you don't like what you see, just change your perception of it. Monaism!" she sang out louder than I would have liked.

"Are you really going to make this about me now? Do you seriously think this place is awesome, and I am the one with the problem?"

"Well, you are the one in the hospital bed. So, yes, if you don't like it here, then you do have a problem. You need the medication going into your arm right now, and the insurance company will only pay for it if you are here in critical condition, which, by the way, you are. I'm thinking that it would be better in the long run, physically and emotionally, to get through this experience without it leaving any long-lasting trauma. How you perceive it here is up to you, but I recommend that you try to make it as pleasant as possible, or you will be miserable. Of course, you could just pout. Your choice."

Tears of anger and frustration filled my eyes. "I just don't get it. How could an insurance company as big as Aetna stop paying for my medicine and not care if I live or die? And how can anyone change their perception about this place? I'm stuck with an apathetic insurance company and a "murse" who hates me. I'm in the middle of a really noisy floor, where the people around me are all half dead. I can't get any rest, so I feel half dead, too. It seems pretty cut and dry to me."

Listening to myself, I realized how much anger I felt, more towards my situation than my surroundings. That anger probably wasn't doing much to improve my health or mental state or the attitude of those around me.

"That's how *you* see it. The way I see it is that you are in the middle of the universe. You are the center of attention, and you have all the floor staff at your beck and call, especially since everyone else around you is, well, sleeping . . . quite soundly. Oh, and someone else is doing the laundry and dishes at home for now; and they'll handle them for at least another week after you get out of here. How's that for perception, baby!"

Her interpretation of my situation did sound better than my pitiful, self-absorbed version. She stared deeply into my eyes as if daring me to start whining again. I decided to adjust my attitude, at least while she was there, and find out if it was possible to make the situation livable. "So how do I respond to this new perception?"

"You can stop calling Dick your 'murse,' for starters. Male nurses don't like that. I imagine he would like a little positive attention from a woman for a change. He is probably not very comfortable socially or he wouldn't prefer working with unconscious patients, not to mention he is a fifty-year-old heterosexual who has never been married. And have you gotten to know the rest of the folks working around here? They are wonderful people."

"When did you meet the staff?" Man, she worked fast.

"When I walked in, I looked them all in the eye and called them by name. This is a tough job, and everyone can use a little appreciation."

"So I should complain less and smile more? And that will get me what?"

"A better experience. Not just for them but for you. We can change our biochemistry just by being happy instead of miserable, no matter the circumstances. Happiness and misery take the same amount of energy. We get to choose which one to feed."

I wasn't ready to let go of my little pity party yet, even if it was to my detriment. Sensing that I was fighting the concept, she continued. "It's always better to deal with the here and now, but remember that belief is stronger than truth."

"I know that Monaism. 'Belief is stronger than truth, unless you believe the truth.' But the truth is that as much as I need my IV medicine, this place sucks."

She laughed. "Well, how about we focus on the first part of that saying. If your belief is strong enough, you can make it a truth, too. It's like that 'if you build it, they will come' theory. If you believe in something with your whole being, even temporarily, you can create an entire world for yourself that is livable. Prisoners do it all the time when locked up in inhumane situations. It keeps them sane. You just have to remember it's for a short time and for a specific reason so that you don't get lost in it. It is called a survivor skill. People only get messed up when they stay in a false reality and don't return to the truth when it's over."

"So you mean I can create my own little version of my time here just by acting the part?"

"You bet! I did it when I was in the hospital dealing with my own medical issues. You will be surprised what a little joy and laughter bring to places like this. I don't think they get much of those here."

"Agreed. But I don't think anything is going to warm up my nurse."

"So? It's not about him; it's about how you are with him. You want to make sure you don't get upset. That could make you sicker, and you will have a harder time breathing. If you don't like what he is saying, try keeping it light. Use humor and love to get your needs met. There are a lot of people on this floor. If it doesn't work with him, then try it with someone else here."

I was too tired to think. "So how do I start this process?"

"Watch and learn, peanut."

With a swing of her hand, she swept my curtain wide as if opening her show on Broadway. She raised the other hand to her brow and called, "Garçon! Garçon! Wherefore art thou?"

Dick walked toward Mona, frowning. "Did you just call me a waiter in French?"

"Oh, yes. There you are, my dear man. My friend here is parched and desperately needs a glass of water. I, of course, reminded her how busy you are, but she does look a little dehydrated, and I can tell that you are on top of your game here at this hospital. I'll bet you have won a few awards for your amazing nursing ability, haven't you? And so good looking to boot."

I felt nauseous. Then I saw the glimmer in his eye.

"Well, as a matter of fact, I did win something a few years ago! I was in the elevator with a man who had a heart attack. He wasn't even a patient, but I brought him back to life while still caring for my patient, who was with us!"

She smiled. "Such valiance and compassion! You just skyrocketed to fame in my book!"

Dick grinned like a little boy and then dropped his head as if he was about to kick a rock. "Well, gosh, thanks for asking. Now, what did you want?"

"Water, love?"

"Sure, I'll be right back."

She turned to me and winked.

"Did you just work that guy, you little manipulator?" I asked, shaking my head in mock criticism.

After he brought my water, Mona sat in the more comfortable chair he'd brought for her. "Of course not! That would be insincere. We all have something interesting and lovable in us somewhere, and it's dying to get out. I believe we can find that something in every human on this planet. We all want to be seen deeply. It's a soul-to-soul connection we are looking for, even if we don't know it."

I had my doubts. "Don't you have to have a soul first?"

That's when I got the look, the one parents give their children when they aren't being polite to guests. "Just as we all had mothers at some point, we all have souls. Some souls are buried under more pain and suffering than others."

Dick stuck his head in and asked, "Mona, is there anything else I can get for you or Lisa before I go on break?"

Wait, did he just call me Lisa?

She looked at me with a twinkle in her eye. "Anything you want?"

I shook my head in disbelief.

She turned back to him. "No, baby, but thanks for asking. You are spectacular, and I will leave today knowing that my friend is in the best of hands. If not, I'm going to have to come after you!" Her smile showed us both that the last part was said in jest.

"Don't you worry. We will take great care of Lisa. She is one of our favorite patients."

With that, he was gone. I turned to her.

"Do you think he will take 'Combative Patient' off my chart now?"

"He will if you stop fighting him and work with what you have in front of you. Like I said before, belief is stronger than truth. If you have to go into survivor mode, which is where you are right now, make up something more fun. Have everyone else play along, too. It helps to look a little deeper than the surface. In Dick's case, he became a nurse for a reason. We just had to help him remember that reason and see him for who he wants to be rather than who he has become. We can create a new reality from anything. Even if it is just for a little while."

"Okay, let me see if I understand this. If I look around and see pure hell here, I can make it into a little game to survive it. If something doesn't work one way, I try another. Also, I need to look for the good, soulful part of every person. Even when I have doubts, I have to remember if a person is breathing, there is a heart in there somewhere. I just have to believe that, and it will come true?"

"And you work from there. Go on, my ace student."

"I can't fake this, because it would be insincere, and they will pick up on that. I have to genuinely care for people and who they are. It helps to see them as the little children they once were instead of the people they have become. And as far as my environment goes, since I can't change it, I have to make it fun in my head. The loud respirators are music, and the bad food is fun to play with . . . like Play Dough. I can always call my husband to bring me something else. The bedpans . . . I'll have to work on that one. Wait! Every time I pee, Dick has to clean it up! The point is to relax and make the experience entertaining instead of getting upset by it all."

"Exactly. Well, my job here is done. I'll let you get some rest and see you again soon. I love you, my little beam of sunshine!"

She floated out of sight, disappearing behind the curtain. I think even the comatose patients could feel her warmth in the ICU. Some energies are so strong you can feel them from across the room because of the negative juju they contain, but Mona's came from a lighter, more spiritual dimension.

She was right. By day three, I had the system wired. Well, at least I didn't hate it there anymore. I smiled as I faked taking unnecessary medication. Maybe that wasn't on the up and up, but it was easier than fighting it. I gave my intubated neighbors names and made up fabulous stories about their lives. Gladys to the left of me (not her real name) ended up there because she was injured during a trapeze performance at the circus and hurt her neck. She would be fine in no time and walk again with a bit of physical therapy. My little bed surrounded by curtains was the fort I always wanted as a child, and I made amazing sculptures with the mashed potatoes I was served for breakfast, lunch, and dinner. Even Dick was impressed with them. The staff was warm and friendly, too, which was a nice change.

One afternoon, Dick strolled in with a big smile and a box. "Who's your buddy?" he asked.

"Well, you, of course. What's in the box?"

He opened it with a flourish. Inside was a bedside commode. Finally strong enough to get out of bed myself, I no longer had to pee in a pan only half the size it should be.

"Oh, Dick! I couldn't love you any more than I do now. Do you think your wife will be jealous?" At that point, I meant every word. I would have loved almost anyone who had delivered a bedside commode to me.

He smiled shyly. "I'm not married, but I hope your husband doesn't mind."

Wow. Mona was right. What's that saying? Fake it until you make it? I was really starting to like this guy and his cute little mannerisms.

"Dick, what am I going to do without you? My husband will never measure up."

"Just know that if you ever have another problem, I will be here to help you get through it. All you have to do is ask for Dick."

I let that one go.

"Thanks, Dick. I will miss you when I go home." I really meant it.

By the time my stay was over, I understood that my primary issue with the hospital had been the fear of returning to it. The anger

I'd projected was more for the heartless insurance company that would rather see me die than pay for life-sustaining medication . . . and the fact that I was sick in the first place.

Mona had helped me understand how to face my fears in one of the worst possible hospital situations I had been in and overcome them, which brought some peace. By keeping my center and my sense of humor, I had learned that I could feel amazing emotionally even when I felt terrible physically. I left thinking that no matter what I was forced to endure, I had the skill to process through it with grace and maybe even a laugh or two.

CHAPTER 26

I personally think we developed language because of our deep need to complain.
Lily Tomlin

FINALLY HOME AND AMONG the living, I gradually settled into my normal routine . . . whatever normal was. My weekly sessions with Mona typically began at 8:30 in the morning. It was like expecting to go for a little car ride after rising and being shot from a cannon instead. I never knew where I would land, but a lot of energy accompanied every touchdown.

One day, she greeted me in her usual cheery manner. "Good morning, sunshine! How are we doing today?"

No one should be that bubbly so early. I certainly wasn't. At least not before a little caffeine.

"Good morning, Mona. What do you want to talk about today?"

"That's entirely up to you. I'm here to listen."

Yeah, right.

"We have been learning so much from your dreams these days. Have you been keeping your dream journal up to date?"

I pulled a tattered notebook out of my purse. Half a leftover peanut butter and jelly sandwich tumbled onto the floor. We both ignored it as I swept it back inside.

"I have. I also looked at some old notebooks and found dreams I'd written down a long time ago. I guess I've been cataloguing my dreams much longer than I thought."

"Great! Anything interesting from last night?"

I flipped through the pages. My dreams seemed so powerful in the moment, but they tended to fade away as the day moved on. I should write them down sooner.

My outlook brightened as I dug through my purse again. "Oh, I remember now! I wrote this one on the back of a magazine cover. I couldn't find my notebook in the dark and didn't want to wake my husband to look for it. It was about a baby again. Why do I keep dreaming about babies?"

"I don't know. Maybe you do, though. Go on."

"I was in a restaurant with this baby. She was sitting in my lap and eating. Then she got sad and began to cry. I tried to console her, but I couldn't figure out what was wrong. After a moment, she stopped crying and started laughing. I felt so relieved. Then she grew sad again. I tried to rock her to sleep, but she popped up and played with something. I think it was a rattle. She hurt her finger and cried again, so I rocked her until she calmed down and went back to being happy. It took a lot of energy to control that baby and keep her calm. It was exhausting."

"Well, what do you think of all that?"

I considered her question briefly before responding. "I think I'm a bad babysitter." It was still early and I hadn't had my tea yet.

"Anything else?" She had such patience with me.

"The baby didn't judge her feelings; she simply let them fly. A child can have a total meltdown over something she wants simply because she can. I would love to do that sometime. Wouldn't it be fun to let yourself freak out when you are tired or frustrated and then go for ice cream?"

"And why don't you?"

"If I did, I would be locked up or medicated, probably both, in the blink of an eye." That one was pretty easy.

"Correct. And why is that? I'll tell you why. In this society, we are taught to control our emotions and even to deny them. What would happen if we simply felt our emotions and didn't judge them?"

"I don't know. Maybe we would feel them and move on to the next thing, the way the baby did."

"Exactly! Look at the brilliance of your dream! Of course, it's important to work through our feelings in a healthy, safe way and not pass our negativity on to those around us. You don't want to project them but process through those emotions instead."

"Project?"

"Sure. It happens all the time. If you feel angry, it's not helpful to yell at someone to get your anger out. That just makes them angry, too. Instead, you can work through the issue by getting the emotion out of your body and understanding what you are feeling in a constructive way."

"That's what I've been doing with the pillow-hitting thing that we use for anger rinsing, right?"

"Exactly. But we've talked about this before. What else is in there?"

"In where?" I preferred being a little ahead of the game. Clearly, that didn't happen very often.

She began watering her plants. "The dream, silly. What else do you see?"

After pondering the question for a minute, I'd come up with nothing. "I dunno. Can you throw me a bone?"

"Okay. What was the last thing you felt in your dream?"

"Exhausted?"

Spinning around, she spilled the contents of her watering can in my lap. "That's right! Why were you exhausted?"

"Because I was trying really hard to comfort a baby who didn't want comfort?"

She handed me a towel to mop up the puddle of water soaking into my skirt. "You're doing that thing again."

"What?"

"Answering all my questions with questions. Why do you do that?"

"Because I am guessing at the answers?"

"You know the answers, but let me help you a bit. You were exhausted because you were working to make someone else happy. You were trying to control what someone else was feeling. It's a little different with a baby, of course, but maybe the message is in the saying 'you can only please some of the people some of the time.' By trying to be a pleaser and make sure everyone is happy, you are losing yourself in the process and wearing your body out. Isn't that part of the disease you have? You feel exhausted all the time?"

"Yes, but do you really believe codependency is part of the reason I got sick?"

"I don't know why you got sick. You will drive yourself crazy if you keep trying to figure it out, so you might want to let the *why* go. Besides, my sense is that there is more than one reason. What's more pressing is to learn a better way to process through these situations. Worrying about what other people think brings us nothing but stress. And no matter how healthy our bodies are, prolonged stress will eventually break us down on a molecular level."

Her message rang true. "I understand what you are saying, but how do I not care about what others think of me?"

"That's the easy part. Just stop judging."

I laughed. "If not judging is the easy part, what's the hard part?"

"The hard part is realizing you are not going to grow if you are stuck in judgment. You will trap yourself in this muck forever unless you learn how to let it go."

"But I don't really care about what people do."

"I'm not talking about judging another. You kill yourself spiritually and emotionally when you judge yourself as not good enough or too different from others. The need to make sure everyone around you is happy will make you miserable, because it is an impossible goal. Let you be you and let them be them and accept everyone for who they are. That will put far less stress on you and your body in the end."

I felt tears welling in my eyes. Again.

"But I can't help feeling like a total failure. I've failed my kids by not being the mom I wanted to be. Being sick all the time means I don't have the energy to do the things I want us to do together. I feel that I've failed on all fronts. I can't work. I can't be a good wife. I can't do anything except lie in bed half the time and watch the world turn without me."

She gently took my hand. "Do you realize what all the pressure you are putting on yourself is doing to your stress level? I'm no doctor, but my guess is that it can't be helping, especially with your particular disease."

I swabbed the puddle of tears that made my lap almost as wet as the watering can had. "You're right. My doctor said that stress is the worst thing for me. But how do I stop stressing? The fact that I'm not there for my kids is killing me."

She jumped up. "Exactly!"

"Exactly what?"

"You are correct. The judgment you have of not being good enough is, indeed, killing you. Stop it."

"That's your advice? Stop it?"

"Yep, that's it. And that's why I get paid the big bucks. I point out the obvious. But this is a big one. Your abilities may have changed, but who knows what incredible lessons your family has learned as a result of those changes. When I met your children the last time you were at the hospital, I saw a level of compassion and understanding in their eyes that most people never reach. And your husband has softened around those crusty edges of his, too.

We can't know how the lives of those around us have changed because of our situation or actions, but don't view change as a bad thing. God can use nearly anything for good. However, if we judge change as bad and create our world from that perspective, we push God out of the picture. Life can feel pretty hopeless when we do that. Is that what you want?"

I slumped in my chair. "No. I suck at playing God no matter how hard I've tried. I do understand what you are talking about, but it is a lot harder than it sounds. Still, I'm willing to give it a try. If I change my perspective and become more accepting of myself and my situation, maybe that will help me accept and love others more, as well."

"And . . .

"And . . . it might help me to stop working so hard at life, which could leave me more energy for other things, like my health. Right?"

"That's right. And by being more relaxed, you will find that others relax more around you. We all have a chance to find the lessons God wants to show us in our lives; we just have to look, some a little harder than others. It is where the magic happens."

"This all makes sense. I have spent so much time fighting for my health that the petty stuff I used to freak out over seems sort of insignificant. When I'm tired, I'm less of a stress case and don't micromanage."

"Yes! See what we can accomplish in a single hour? Remember, if you do not learn and own the lesson of your struggle, you can get stuck in the struggle. Monaism 103."

"Right. Got it. I think."

"Oh, don't worry. You will never get *it*."

"Why do you keep telling me that?"

"Hopefully, we never stop learning. Ever. So we won't completely get it, because *it* will always be something new and magical."

"Got it. Or not."

I left Mona's office wondering if I was acquiring a better grip on reality or losing my grip altogether. Sometimes I felt like Alice in Wonderland talking to the Mad Hatter. I wasn't sure which side of the looking glass we were on.

CHAPTER 27

All the art of living lies in a fine mingling of letting go and holding on.
Henry Ellis

I WAS LATE FOR MY WEEKLY coffee date with the girls. It had been a particularly rough morning for me physically, and I struggled to get ready. When I arrived, I noticed the mood wasn't as jovial as usual. Ours was typically not a serious group, so the low energy in the room took me by surprise.

I decided to ignore it. "Hey, guys, what's up?"

Maude turned to me, her eyes blazing with anger. "What's up? I'll tell you what's up! The world has gone mad, and the children of today have gone to hell and are never coming back. That's what's up!"

Usually, I found Maude's sense of the dramatic refreshing, but she seemed genuinely upset.

"Did something happen to the world's children that I missed?"

I had been a little preoccupied with my health, after all.

For a minute, I thought her head might explode. "Did something happen? Yes, something happened! Last night I was leaving the mall, and a kid ran up and grabbed my purse in the parking lot. My Dolce & Gabbana purse! You know, the brown one . . . not the black one I got last summer in Paris."

"Not the big bag!" Gabby often borrowed the big bag from Maude.

Annoyed, she responded, "No, the little one with the metal clasps on the side. Anyway, it was a nightmare. I had to give a report to a mall cop who was half my age, which made me late for my bridge game. I don't even think he was a real policeman."

"Of course he wasn't a real policeman. If he was a real policeman, he wouldn't be working in a mall." Cheryl was the voice of reality in our group.

"Anyway!" Maude wasn't about to let anyone steal her big moment. "I was walking to my car, and this guy just appears from the shadows and demands that I give him my purse! Just like that. He couldn't be any older than my Luke."

"Isn't Luke, like, seventeen?" Gabby asked as she leaned in for the creamer.

"He will be in the fall. But he would never in a million years think of doing anything so horrible. What kind of monster steals an innocent woman's purse as she is leaving Saks?"

"Drug crazed?" Cheryl asked, while swallowing her morning medications with her latte.

I couldn't resist offering my two cents, as well. "Maybe he needed it more than you."

I swear I saw a light bulb glow above Minnie's head after I spoke. "I just had the kids read *Les Misérables* as their English assignment, and we saw the play for art class. Jean Valjean, the lead character, is just a boy when he steals a loaf of bread from the market to feed his starving family. He is sent to prison for five years of hard labor. When he's caught trying to escape, another ten years was added on."

Minnie homeschooled her four children, and she came up with some interesting educational activities.

"Why are you telling us this, Minnie?" Maude was getting annoyed again.

"My point is that maybe the boy who stole your purse was hungry or needed the money for his family. When he saw you with all your purchases from Saks Fifth Avenue and your expensive car, he could have thought you didn't need your bag as much as he needed the money in it. He might have taken it so his family could eat or pay their rent. Money is pretty tight these days. And unemployment is at an all-time high."

I tossed in another two cents. "Or maybe he is a runaway who was kicked out of the house by his mother's drunk boyfriend. He probably has nowhere to live and needed money for some type of shelter."

"I'm sticking with the idea that he needed the money for drugs."
It probably made Cheryl feel better to know that other people were
taking them, as well.

Maude slammed her cup on the table. "Hello! Is anyone going to
ask me how I am? Don't you care about what a horrible situation it
was for me? I am the victim here and will have to suffer with this
memory for the rest of my life."

Her shoulders slumped as the weight of the experience crashed
upon them. I thought I even saw a tear in her eye, but then my
attention shifted to Minnie when she offered a different perspective.

"In our class on world religion, I taught my kids that many
cultures believe there are no accidents. They say that while still in
the realm of Spirit, we decide the lessons we will pursue here. Then
Spirit helps us master those lessons by creating the conditions
necessary for us to receive our chosen experience. Or there is another
option. Possibly, it was karma."

Minnie tended to have an unusual take on every situation. I
didn't always agree with her perceptions, but they offered me a fresh
perspective to consider.

Maude was staring blankly at Minnie. "And karma is . . . ?"
Apparently, her interest had been piqued.

"Karma is the Buddhist and Hindu belief in the process of cause
and effect. If you do A, B will happen. If you plant tomato seeds and
then water and tend them, tomatoes will grow. Or as the Bible says,
'Whatsoever a man soweth, that shall he also reap.' I think St. Paul
said that in the book of Galatians."

"Do you honestly believe I did something awful, and now I am
paying the price by being robbed?" Maude's curiosity was quickly
turning to anger.

Minnie put her hand on Maude's arm to reassure her. "No, of
course not. And I'm not saying it is okay to steal or hurt someone
else by your actions. I'm saying that things happen for a reason, and
there may be a lesson in it for you. Unspeakable, horrible things
happen to people. I don't believe it is because they are bad people or
they need to be punished. I do think everything that crosses our path
may contain a lesson, though. We have to choose whether to accept
the lesson and grow from it or become a victim to it. What happens
from then on depends on our perspective."

"What do you mean?" Cheryl apparently didn't like where the conversation was going. She had been mourning her husband ever since he left. Her game plan for getting out of her funk was limited to the bottle of wine she drank every night and the antidepressants she took regularly.

Minnie elaborated. "Life isn't supposed to be fair. I believe it is meant to be a classroom, like homeschooling my kids. I take everything we do and try to turn it into a teaching moment for them. My hope is that they will become more conscious of what they do and see life as a quest for wisdom."

I was struck by the synchronicity of life. It was as if Mona had spoken to the group through Minnie. It helped me with what she and I had talked about in our last session.

A little cynicism was evident in Maude's voice when she replied. "School 24/7. Your house must be a barrel of fun to hang out in."

"It is, actually. We view everything as an adventure. We don't get caught up in drama, because we don't become victims to our circumstances. Instead, we try to understand the various aspects of a situation and discover our part in it. Our goal is to learn from everything we do, which should help the kids think for themselves and grow accordingly."

That struck a nerve with me. "So what you are saying is that no matter what happens, from a violent crime to a horrible illness, life isn't black and white, and there are many ways to look at the same situation?"

Minnie looked relieved that I had chimed in. "Yes! And we can look at anything from another person's vantage point as easily as our own. It helps us be more understanding, which makes it easier to understand whatever it is we are supposed to learn."

I considered the concept she was trying to convey. "All right, we can use Maude's situation as an example. Let's say we found out that kid was desperate for money because his family was poor, like Valjean's in *Les Mis*. The kid stole Maude's purse to put food on the table. She has many purses and lives an affluent lifestyle. Her lesson could be . . ."

I had to come up with something positive or Maude might throw her coffee at me. Before anything came to mind, Maude said quietly, "Compassion?"

I hadn't seen that coming.

Minnie's eyes softened. "Exactly, Maude. Compassion. And maybe he is supposed to get caught for his own lesson about taking from others. Who knows? There are probably a hundred more scenarios we could propose for the situation. At the end of the day, it isn't about the other person. It is about us and what we are learning in the process."

I thought about all the physically sick people in the world. So many of us become victims of our illnesses and never truly grasp the lessons they were intended to teach. Especially me. Maybe Mona was right and it was time to forgive myself for getting sick. Perhaps I needed to work on understanding what I was to learn instead of focusing on my inadequacies.

We all have difficult situations that play out in our lives. Wouldn't it be great if we could figure out what we are supposed to learn rather than living under the shadow of our challenges? My biological father used to tell me that he did the things he did because he'd had a horrible childhood and his father abused him. Child abuse is inexcusable, but, unfortunately, it is not uncommon. If that is the case, we have to choose whether to get stuck in the abuse and pass it on to someone else or take the time to mourn, learn, and grow from the experience. Choosing the high road isn't easy, but with a little help and a great desire to change, it is possible.

Maude spoke again. "So you are saying that we can't change other people; we can only change ourselves. If I keep focused on me and how I want to react to the world, I don't become a victim to it; I'm just part of it. Sounds great, but I think I rather like getting mad and filing a report. It makes for a better story."

The serious look on her face told me she wasn't joking. I tried not to roll my eyes, as that would be judging. However, I couldn't keep from feeling a little frustrated by what I viewed as her self-serving attitude. "It's your journey, Maude."

Minnie smiled. "How's that saying go? Hurting people hurt people? What happens to us is just part of our experience. How we handle it is what makes us who we are. The best part is that we get to choose who we want to be. Nobody takes that away from us. Lisa is right. It is your choice, and there is nothing wrong with following through with a police report; accountability is equally important. All I am saying is that whatever you do, do it with awareness."

It reminded me of my own circumstances. "Coming off a long hospital stay, it is easy to feel angry about my situation and be nasty to those around me because of it. After all I've gone through, haven't I earned the right to be really mad? Probably. However, if I'm angry, I just create more anger around me. Then I end up becoming a victim to their negative attitude towards me, an attitude for which I am partially responsible."

Maude appeared to be a little lost. "What?"

"It's pure physics. We get back what we put out. Like Minnie said before, terrible things happen . . . horrible things for some, and my compassion for them is huge. But we all get to decide what we are going to do with our experiences and how we are going to be in the world in spite of them. At the end of the day, sitting in anger only hurts me more and causes more stress on my body. So what's the point of staying mad?"

Maude took a sip of her latte before she replied. "That is a great concept, but don't you think it is a little idealistic? How are we supposed to do that?"

It was Gabby's turn to offer an example. "I was dealing with some old stuff in my life that I couldn't shake for a while, and it kept coming up again and again. It drove me crazy until I sat back and took stock of my life. I got tired of blaming everyone else for what was going on in my world and decided I needed to take action to break the cycle. It was very empowering."

Cheryl had been listening intently. "And you did this how?"

Gabby took a slow, deep breath. "I started by reading a couple of self-help books that caught my eye. Then I began journaling. I wrote crazy stuff, like letters to people who had wronged me. I wrote to tell them how much I hated them."

Maude cut in. "You sent letters to them? Isn't that just passing on the abuse?"

"Of course not. I didn't send them; I just wrote them to get the thoughts and feelings out of my head and body. Some of the things I wrote were so absurd and filled with such grossness that they made me laugh. I also drew terrible pictures and cried a lot. It helped get the ball rolling, but after I was done, I needed a little more help."

I thought about how it would feel to send hate letters to all those I felt had wronged me in the past. Then I contemplated the feeling of receiving letters from those who felt I had hurt them. I suspected the quantities of incoming and outgoing letters would be nearly equal. We humans tend to remember the instances when have been hurt, but we are quick to forget when we hurt others. I decided to lay down my mental pen and refocus my attention on the conversation.

"So what did you do?"

I wondered if Gabby would come clean about her therapy sessions.

She focused on her coffee cup. "I looked into a few 12-step programs. You would be surprised how many different kinds there are. Some of them were helpful, but I felt that I needed more personalized attention. So I went another direction."

Maude looked shocked. "What direction was that?"

"One of personal growth. I never looked back."

The roads to empowerment are as individual as we are. Our job is to find the one that works best for us. Looking around the table, I felt so proud of those women. We were all moving forward at our own speeds, but we were moving just the same.

Situations in my life were becoming clearer, too. It was as if I was sitting on top of the world and looking down, watching myself while I was still in my own movie. Almost dying multiple times hadn't been the easiest way to change my outlook, but it was certainly effective. Overcoming huge challenges makes the world seem less petty. The small stuff no longer mattered as much. Being sick had forced me to keep my eye on the big picture and what truly matters.

As hard as it was spending half my life sick, I was grateful for the wisdom that came with it.

CHAPTER 28

A poem begins in delight and ends in wisdom.

Robert Frost

AS I WALKED INTO MONA'S office for what felt like the millionth time, I thought about my latest epiphany and how similar insights occurred on a regular basis after our sessions. It was as if Mona planted seeds in my head, which I watered and tended throughout the week.

Of course, once those seeds germinated, I took full credit for my revelations, throwing them out to her as fabulous new ideas direct from my brain. Her response was always the same.

"Oh, honey, that's brilliant! Look at the wisdom!"

The process continued for months, until I looked back at my notes and realized most of my big ideas were the gems she had offered me repeatedly over time. Guess I wasn't as smart as I thought. When I asked why she didn't start each session with "I told you so," her answer was simple.

"Why should I take credit for your knowledge? I am just a guide to help you find your inner truth. You have to own your truths or they won't stick. If I tell you something and it doesn't drop in permanently, nothing will change. It will just get stuck in your left brain, and you would only recall the thing but not feel it. If you come up with the idea on your own, with a little help from me, it's yours forever, because you experienced it."

Maybe her answer wasn't all that simple, but I understood her point.

"You mean it is the difference between reading about some beautiful vacation spot versus being there in person?"

"Yes! You don't fully understand or comprehend the majesty of anything until you experience it."

"And you are totally okay with your clients plagiarizing your ideas?" I couldn't imagine anyone being all right with that.

"It happens all the time. They say to me, 'I had a revelation the other day, Mona! I figured out blah blah blah, and I learned blah, blah blah, and I did it all by myself!'"

"And you let them get away with that?"

"What do I care how they learn something, as long as they learn it and become better people as a result. I consider it an honor that they get what I am saying and change because of it."

"I'll keep that in mind the next time I lecture the kids."

We sat in stillness for a moment. It was odd. Her office was rarely quiet, and the energy level was seldom as low as it was then. Mona stared into what seemed like another dimension, lost in thought. She then turned to me and asked in a softer, more soulful voice than I had ever heard from her, "Have I told you my favorite Monaism?"

"No, tell me."

"The only way to keep your gifts is to give them all away."

"And that means . . . ?"

"You will figure it out soon enough, love."

"Why, is something going to happen?"

"I don't know. Maybe. Remember this: no matter what happens, you have the skills and resources to handle anything that comes. You just need to ask for guidance when you need it."

"Are you quitting me or something?"

"No, baby, but I won't always be here either."

Her behavior made me uneasy. It was as if I was only seeing half the picture she saw. "Okay, but we have a session next week. There's a lot to cram into my little brain, and I am committed to getting this body back on track one way or another."

"I know you are, and I'm sure you will . . . one way or another."

She was a funny one. Always talking as if she was five pages ahead of the chapter I was reading.

As I drove home, I thought about how grateful I was for the experience of working with someone who completely understood me and what I was going through. As an added bonus, she never let me get away with anything. One of Mona's favorite Monaisms was "You can't change someone else; you can only change you with them." She had certainly changed me with . . . well . . . everyone. Especially me with me.

I used to feel bad about all the things I couldn't do, even before I got sick. If I ran a marathon, I would kick myself for not running it faster. After my latest hospital stay, I was thrilled to be able to walk around the block. Seriously. I high-fived my neighbors like a four-year-old during an hour-long stroll that should have taken ten minutes. I was deliriously happy to be out of my wheelchair instead of killing myself for landing there in the first place. Mona had helped me change my relationship with me. She illustrated how to be self-compassionate and forgiving by accepting all my strengths and weaknesses. I also found that the more I directed compassion and forgiveness to myself, the more I felt them for others.

The world might be transformed if we all gave those gifts to ourselves. Lord knows, we all mess up. Why not learn from our mistakes and let them go without all the judgment we usually plop on top of our heads.

I thought of the many people in my life who could benefit from some Mona time. I might not be able to change them, and I wouldn't want to try. But she sure could.

CHAPTER 29

Smells like burning bridges.
Train

THE REST OF THE WEEK was relatively uneventful, but I kept thinking about what I was learning and how some of my friends would benefit from a few sessions with my dear therapist, as well. Pulling into the parking lot to meet them, I decided to bring up the subject and inquire about any interest they might have. I was growing because of the lessons she was teaching me and wanted that for them, too.

Sipping my cup of courage (that is, coffee), I settled on the soft approach. Taking a deep breath, I said, "This may sound strange, but have any of you noticed something different about me lately?"

Maude stared at me without expression. "Did you have some work done?"

"No."

She tried again. "Your hair is fabulous!"

Why do people immediately look to the hair when figuring out what's changed?

"I haven't taken my hair out of this ponytail all week, Maude, but thanks. I mean, do I seem different personality wise?"

Gabby looked at me intently before answering. "You seem a lot more . . . I don't know. Peaceful? No. Accepting? Maybe. Wait! I think you appear more integrated."

That wasn't what I was going for, but whatever. "Integrated, Gabby? What do you mean?"

"Before, you seemed happy on the outside but kind of sad on the inside. When you got sick, you seemed sad on the outside but more peaceful on the inside. Now your insides and your outsides match."

I wasn't sure what I should do with that analysis. "Are my insides and outsides happy or sad now?"

"Neither. Both. If you are sad on the inside, you move it through to the outside, so it goes away faster. If you are happy on the inside, your light shines brightly on the outside, as well. You flow through life more and are easier to read. Like an open book. It's nice, because I sometimes felt as if I was walking on eggshells with you. I could never figure out what mood you were in. Now you feel more honest and real. "

I'd appreciated Gabby more and more since her "friend" started working with Mona. Her light was shining more brightly, too, and it was great that she no longer needed antidepressants.

Cheryl took a long, critical survey of me. "Yeah, I kind of get that, too. You are more talkative about things you notice but not in a judgmental way. If you are asked for your opinion, you call it as you see it from your perspective, but you aren't righteous or anything. It feels safer to talk to you."

I hadn't realized I'd been considered unsafe to talk to or as moody as Gabby had mentioned, but I was glad they were feeling more comfortable with me. I felt more comfortable with me, too. However, the discussion was veering off track.

I switched to a more direct course. "I was thinking about everything I have learned since I began to study with Mona. I wondered if any of you were interested in learning some new processing skills by working with her, too."

I held my breath as I waited for someone to say something. No one said a word. You could hear a pin drop.

The silence continued for so long that I began to compose a plan to deflect my question. That way they would forget I asked. I was formulating an idea to fake breathing trouble or a heart attack; maybe they would take pity on me and call the paramedics. If I held my breath long enough, there was a chance I could pass out. Would that be easier than the deafening silence?

Most definitely.

Gabby was the first to speak. "Um, when was the last time you talked to Mona?"

"Last week. Why?"

She stared into her coffee cup as she said, "You really loved working with her."

What do you say when someone states the obvious? "Sure. She has helped me understand why I do the things I do and how to change the stuff that is really annoying about me. She has also shown me how to deal more effectively with stress; she can do that for each of you, too, if you are interested."

Gabby squirmed in her chair like a little girl before glancing up from her latté. "No. She can't."

Maybe inviting the group to study with Mona hadn't been as good an idea as I originally thought. I knew Gabby was working with her, even if she was doing so secretly. Were her sessions not progressing as well as mine had?

I should have kept my mouth shut. I hate learning lessons by looking stupid.

Gabby stirred the long-dissolved sugar in her drink with wild abandon. Maude fixated on her shoes. Finally, Gabby spoke quietly. "I am so sorry that I have to tell you this, but Mona is dead."

Disbelief flooded through me. *Surely, she said Mona is fed. What does she care if she eats or not? Or was it that she was in bed?* None of it made sense to me. My mind swirled out of control as I listened to the beating of my heart. *Surely she didn't say Mona is dead. Not possible. It hasn't been that long since our last meeting, and she wouldn't do that to me. Do that to me? What am I thinking?*

It was a good thing my insides and outsides didn't match at that moment. If they had, the numerous thoughts and feelings revolving through my head might have made my friends so dizzy they'd feel like throwing up. I certainly wanted to.

My voice was barely above a whisper when I asked, "What?"

She slowly continued. "There was a car accident. A tire blew out on her way back from the desert, and the car went off an embankment. It rolled, and she was ejected. Mona died instantly. I'm really sorry, honey."

Honey? She can't call me honey! Nobody can call me honey but Mona, and she is dead. How can she be dead? She can't be dead, because I still need her. Everyone still needs her. What will happen now? I am freaking out. Why am I freaking out?

I was freaking out because I didn't know if I could handle life by myself. She was more than my therapist. She was someone who could connect with me on a deeper level. Mona understood me better than anyone, including myself. She explained me to me. How could I possibly process my issues without some help? How would I understand the woman I faced in the mirror every morning, not to mention the rest of the world, without some coaching? Life is hard and heavy, but she walked alongside me, teaching me while making it fun and light. We could laugh, cry, yell, and play at the same time. I hadn't lost just a mentor. I had lost a friend, too. Just like that. I felt completely alone.

Why is this happening?

The world started spinning again. I needed to get out of there and go home to think. I couldn't wait to get to my little closet, where everything felt safer. Could this be a prank to discover if I was ready to go it on my own?

If so, I was clearly failing the test.

CHAPTER 30

ONCE HOME, ALL I COULD do was cry. How could she leave me? What would happen to me without her? I was improving but certainly not finished with the work we were doing. I had become more aware, but there was no enlightenment. That was light years away.

Playing the mental tape of our last session in my mind, I felt sure she had been setting me up for something. Was it her death? Did she know what was coming? How could she have known? It's not as if you plan to have the right rear tire blow out and your car sail off an embankment. Still, our last talk had been kind of strange. I remember her sharing her favorite Monaism: "The only way to keep your gifts is to give them away."

Had she been downloading her work into countless brains to pass it on before she left the planet? What was she thinking by transferring it to mine? She should have picked a better brain, a brain that paid more attention. Was I supposed to help carry on her legacy?

I seriously doubted that.

I wondered what kind of legacy I would leave. My kids might say, "There goes Mom. She was a real pain about picking up our things." Not a stirring memorial.

Note to self: work on a more inspirational legacy.

I felt that the increased strength in my body and the recent consistency in my health were due to a newfound emotional stability, fragile as it was. At least I recognized the underlying stress I'd been carrying from unresolved issues floating around in my head and body. I was terrified to slide backward on a physical or emotional level. How was I supposed to maintain the progress I'd made by myself?

Normally, I would talk it over with Mona, but I was left to figure it out on my own. In the dark recesses of my closet, I curled up in a tiny ball with my journal. It was as if a huge tree had blown over and landed in the middle of the new path we had created together. It was too heavy and overwhelming to shove to the side of the road. Mona had offered me hope for a better tomorrow, one filled with health and happiness. I had no other guides in my life and no one to turn to for help. The brighter new day she'd promised had gotten a lot darker.

Confused and alone, I lay on the floor and cried. Fortunately, the floor was littered with clothes, so I had plenty of options for wiping my tear-streaked face. As I reached for one of my softer t-shirts, I saw an old journal filled with the instructions she had given me for processing through tough times. I started to laugh and flipped it open to read my notes:

When we sit in self-pity, we are looking to be rescued by someone other than ourselves. When we are sad, it's not about others; it's about us figuring ourselves out and taking action. We are simply experiencing our feelings.

Self-pity was a big issue for me at that particular juncture. Reading my notes helped me realize that I was viewing Mona's death from the perspective of how it would affect me. Isn't it interesting how we can turn almost anything around and make it about us? On the other hand, death can easily be about the living and their relationship with the people they lost. Especially when trying to figure out how to grieve. I read on:

It is important to get our feelings out on paper, because when we write, we bypass our left brain and can see clearly where we are emotionally. We can write to a person or about a situation that happened or about any issue we need to let go of. It can also be done repeatedly to delve deeper into the problem. Our subconscious can have more going on than our conscious mind knows. Also, as you write, don't be thrown off by the feeling of finality that comes with the "let go" energy of the letter. What you are releasing is the codependency and bondage, not the person.

I laughed again. Codependency is something I've always struggled with. Only Mona could call me on it from beyond the grave.

In the back of my notes were two letters she used to work through her process. The first presented a method for delving deeper into the reason we are upset. The second was useful for those really bad days. She called it the "Ultimate Fuck You." She'd told me she liked to use the word *fuck* because it had an electrical charge to it, which is helpful for getting the anger out of our bodies. It takes us to the dark side of things so we can release emotions we need to eject, to the point of the absurd, if necessary. Even in death, Mona was still counseling me. That time I didn't fight her and did as she asked.

To start the process, I was to sit in a quiet place with a pen and paper. It had to be somewhere I wouldn't be disturbed so that I could let it flow, as I'd done for the anger work. I followed her instructions carefully.

The Release Letters

Option 1:

Dear (insert name here),

I miss you so much because . . .

I loved you because . . .

I loved me with you because . . .

I need to say good-bye and let go of you because . . .

I am letting go of . . .

This frees me because . . .

It makes me feel . . .

Thank you for teaching me . . .

Because of you, I can be . . .

I love you because . . .

I hate you because . . .

You scared me because . . .

It reminded me of another time when . . .

I feel hurt because . . .

I am sad because . . .

Through this process, I learned . . .

Releasing you is like . . .

And it feels like . . .

I can walk away knowing . . .

I wish . . .

I am better knowing you because . . .

I am so grateful for you teaching me . . .

Option 2:

Fuck you, (insert name here)!

I hate your guts because you did . . .

And made me feel . . .

And I wish your head would explode because . . .

I worked through both letters. There can be so many emotions that twist inside us when we lose someone. They range from sadness to anger, and it's possible to experience several simultaneously. I pulled up all of those feelings and many more. It sounded a little crazy for me to write an anger letter to someone who'd been killed in a car accident, but not judging my feelings helped me cleanse them. My notes reminded me how important it is to understand my own feelings before trying to understand the situation or the other person. Otherwise, I might end up ignoring them. No wonder she called it "The Ultimate Rinse."

I wrote, cried, hit the pillow, and repeated until I was exhausted. Crawling out of my closet hours later, I realized it was up to me to find my own way. Determined to continue my journey, I silently thanked my dear friend for the time we had together and vowed never to forget her or the lessons she'd taught me.

Later that day, as I was cleaning the house, numerous thoughts swirled around in my head. My children had been looking at the old matchbox cars my husband played with when he was a child. As I carefully placed each antique replica back in its designated spot in the carrying case, an idea came to me.

Before I became sick, my mind had resembled that car carrier. Each of my opinions had fit neatly in its labeled slot, and every well-ordered case resided on a hard, inflexible shelf in the back of my brain. Such a rigid environment is important for keeping items of value safe for years in your garage, but it's not ideal when life throws you a curveball and you don't know how to stretch to grab it.

Mona helped me comprehend that our journey isn't neat and organized. It is messy. As soon as you think you've figured it out, life flips itself upside down, and you have to look at it from a different angle. She also helped me understand that we don't have to fear or dread the chaos that happens; we can view it as a fun, sometimes challenging, growth opportunity. I guess the greatest thing she taught me was to trust my inner voice as deeply as I trusted the process she taught . . . and to stay open to new ideas.

In Mona's words, a true miracle is a change in perception. Observing my circumstances through new filters kept me from becoming a victim to them.

Despite the amount of anguish my experiences and illnesses had caused me and my family, the lessons we learned were far too valuable to give up.

Would I recommend my experience to others?

Hell, no.

We all have our own journeys to travel. Some are less painful than others, but they are equally important. If we compare our existence to another's, we lose the context of the lesson, for each is as individual as our own thumbprint. The blueprint for our lives is there for us to uncover so that we will become the people we were meant to be.

As I put the last toy car away, a tear rolled down my cheek. I thought about how many of my perceptions had shattered and been rebuilt on stronger foundations with her help and guidance. The rigid container that held the preconceived ideas about myself and my surroundings had been smashed. I could finally breathe in the fresh air that had always been there outside that box. I knew my journey was not over; it was just turning in a new direction. Fear had been replaced with faith, as I was confident another mentor would come forward if I asked for one and prayed enough.

I decided to start praying.

Hard and often.

BODY

CHAPTER 31

Sometimes, I feel the fear of uncertainty stinging clear,
And I can't help but ask myself how much I let that fear take the wheel and steer.
Incubus

MINNIE CALLED ME the next day. Her voice was tender and soulful. "I'm so sorry for your loss of Mona. I know you two were on a good path together. I noticed that after working with her, the light inside you turned on."

Minnie had taken her kids to a meditation retreat in India the previous summer so they could find their "inner beauty." Her vocabulary hadn't been the same since. Unfortunately, it required translation to regular mom lingo for full comprehension.

"What do you mean?"

"I mean I always saw a glimmer of light glowing in there somewhere, but it was covered up. You've been doing a great job of pulling the covers off and letting it shine. There are other ways of turning up the intensity though."

That wasn't a lot of help in the translation department.

"Thanks, Minnie, but I am not about to start over with another therapist, if that is what you have in mind. It took months for me to fill Mona in on my history; she probably had a file cabinet with volumes of notes detailing all of my issues. It sounds overwhelming, and I seriously doubt I have the strength for it."

She paused, almost as if she'd expected my answer. "But do you have the flexibility?"

"The flexibility? You're still not making any sense."

"I have been going to a yoga class taught by an old friend of ours. We learn all sorts of things about ourselves there and not just about how bendable we are."

I'd read that some people take yoga for spiritual reasons. I tried taking a few classes when I was well but got frustrated and quit because I couldn't touch my toes. I was never a very patient yogi.

"Where are you going with this, Minnie? You know how much I hate yoga."

"You hated yoga when you were healthy and running a lot, because you thought it was a waste of time. You said it wasn't a good workout, so why bother. Remember? Now you are in a different place physically and mentally. Why not give it another try?"

My head ached at the thought of opening myself up to something or someone else. It was too soon. My strength steadily declined as the conversation continued. The only response I could muster was "Why?"

Her reply was like cold water thrown in my face.

"Because you don't really have anything else going for you right now but disease and self-pity. Weren't you the one saying you wanted to change? Maybe this can be a good way of doing that. Also, yoga is a gentle method for connecting your nerves with your muscles and your mind with your body. Isn't that part of the issue with your neuromuscular autoimmune disease? You've become disconnected?"

She had a point. I was feeling very disconnected, but in an overall sense rather than physically. I decided not to decide until my head was clearer. I also needed to feel sorry for myself a little longer. It wasn't the most enlightened approach, but it seemed to feel right in the moment. Then again, those negative feelings might have had something to do with the high dose of steroids the doctor had added to my medication regimen. It was more than I could figure out in the midst of my drug-induced brain fog. The steroids also made my skin feel like it was crawling off my body, so I opted to stay in bed and stop thinking.

Besides, I wouldn't be comfortable working with the instructors I knew. There were several teachers at my old gym, but they taught competitive, judgmental yoga. I had no interest in attending a class where the students try to outdo each other by seeing who can bend the farthest or stand the tallest in a pose.

Minnie could probably sense my anxiety through the phone. "Promise you will consider it with an open mind when you are feeling better. You have come so far, and something out of the box could be just what you need."

Minnie was right. Not being open to the concept at that time didn't mean I wasn't ready at all. Things would probably be more manageable after a nap; they always are. "Okay. I will think about it. But if I were to do yoga, I would have to work with a teacher who has incredible patience. Someone who understands my condition. Otherwise, it could be a total disaster."

She chuckled. "Or a total success. Anything is possible."

I hung up realizing I'd sounded like the old, pessimistic me again. I didn't like that person anymore. Maybe I should try a new approach by staying open to what might come my way.

Who knows what can happen once we are open to new ideas?

CHAPTER 32

The doctor of the future will give no medicine but will interest his patients in diet and the cause and prevention of disease.

Thomas Edison

I DREADED MEETING the girls for coffee more than usual. Bella, a former neighbor I hadn't seen in a while, would be joining us. To say she was a Type A personality would be an understatement. When she lived in my neighborhood, Bella served as chairman of the Junior League and president of the PTA. She was in charge of the school carnival, ran at least three marathons a year, and worked full time in sales. I'm pretty sure she even made her own strawberry preserves.

It was a little ridiculous.

Even Bella's six-pack abs were intimidating, and her hair always looked better than mine, too. Not that I compared or noticed at all. She was one of those people who set impossible standards no one could live up to. When we created shared projects for our children's classroom, her part was always better baked, glued, stapled, stenciled, and/or scrapbooked.

Looking back, I may have been slightly jealous; isn't that the root of envy?

Bella's husband owned his own company, a very successful construction firm. Unfortunately, when the economy fell apart, so did his business. Like a lot of employers in our area, he had to close the doors and lay off all his employees, many of whom were our neighbors and friends. In the process, he was forced to file bankruptcy, both personally and professionally. He and Bella lost their home, their car, and their pride. It was horrible to watch. The family moved in with his parents, who lived across town, while they got back on their feet. They virtually dropped out of sight after pulling out of everything, including the kids' schools.

My heart went out to the family, but I wasn't sure how to convey that. As I was wondering what to say to her when she joined us for coffee, I heard a soft voice from behind me.

"Hi, Lisa. How are you doing?"

I almost didn't recognize her. She wore a long skirt and a t-shirt with a pair of flip-flops. I'd never seen Bella in flip-flops before. Her usually perfectly coiffed hair was pulled back in a casual ponytail, and she wore very little makeup. Her energy had changed to something softer and more peaceful. It was not the crazy, high-stress stuff I'd come to expect. She appeared relaxed, Botox free, and truly beautiful.

I couldn't hide my astonishment at the change in her. "Bella? You look amazing!"

She smiled as she ordered a green tea.

The minute she sat down, Maude launched an interrogation.

"Okay, Bella, what's your secret, because I have never seen you look this good or this happy? Are you having an affair?"

She laughed. "No."

Minnie was next. "Did you hit the lotto?"

"Nope. But that would certainly solve our debt problems."

It was my turn. "Did you marry a younger man? Don't keep us all in suspense. What has happened to you?"

Bella shrugged. "I guess it was yoga."

Almost in unison, we all asked, "Yoga?"

"Yeah. Yoga. When Bill, the kids, and I moved in with my in-laws, I had no idea what to do with myself. I was at the end of my rope. I slumped into a serious depression, gained a bunch of weight, and lost hope. I was miserable but not just because we had lost everything. I was miserable to the core. I felt as if the money and accolades I'd gotten from working on and heading community events had become my identity. Once that was gone, so was I."

She sat calmly, lost in thought, before continuing. "The best word to describe that time is *lost*. Then, a few months ago, I stopped by the YMCA to pick up the kids and accidentally walked into a yoga class. I watched as they finished the class and sat quietly on their mats. The teacher told them a story. Her voice sounded so relaxed and tranquil that I stayed to listen. It changed my life."

My interest was piqued. "What was the story?" I figured any story that is life changing is worth a listen.

For a moment she looked to the sky as if her next words waited somewhere up there. Absently clutching her tea to her chest, she closed her eyes and started slowly, almost whispering.

"It was a beautiful story about a caterpillar that believed she had come into being only to eat and sleep and do what the rest of the caterpillars did. However, she was unhappy, somehow sensing that there was another dimension she had not yet experienced. One day, driven by a strange longing she didn't understand, the caterpillar decided to become still and silent. Hanging from the branch of a tree, she wove a cocoon around her body.

"Although constrained and uncomfortable, she waited inside the cocoon, sensing and aware. Her patience bore fruit, for when the cocoon burst open, she was no longer a lowly worm but a beautiful, resplendent, winged butterfly that dazzled the sky. She soared, no longer limited to a wormlike existence but free and limitless. The caterpillar had been transformed into a thing of air and lightness, magic and beauty.

"Once the transformation had taken place, it was impossible for the butterfly to return to being a worm. In the cocoon, the caterpillar had become one with her inner being and, through this union, she had reached her ultimate nature."

Bella opened her eyes and looked at us. I sat with my mouth open and my mind blank. Everyone around the table wore the same vacant expression. She started to laugh. "Pretty out there, huh?"

I appreciated the new version of Bella a lot more than the one I'd first met. Maybe Minnie had been right after all about my trying yoga with Bella as my teacher.

Bella took another stab at explaining the story. Given the looks on our faces, she could have been dumbing it down for us.

"I realized that my unhappiness was due to the circumstances in my life. It was time for an overhaul. I didn't know the person I had become. I was stuck in my own cocoon, staying hidden for fear that others would see me as damaged. Somehow, I needed to find a way out. For me, that way was yoga. Yoga was my path towards being boundless. It can transform and liberate us so that we can reach an unbounded state."

All of us had been holding our breath as she spoke. Maude was the first to start breathing again. "So you have to get all bound up to be unbounded?" She enjoyed breaking up tense moments with humor.

Bella looked at her with compassion. "Humans, unlike animals, are not merely existing. They are becoming. To evolve as a human being is to become aware of one's limitations and strive with intense passion towards the transcendence for which we all have the potential. So I guess you do have to get bound up to become unbounded, Maude."

She surveyed the table and continued. "At first, yoga supported me by increasing my flexibility and allowing me to keep up with the demands of our new lifestyle. I practiced mostly at home, because the weight I'd gained made me feel uncomfortable in my body. When I made the decision to lose the weight, yoga was there for me. Eventually, yoga's more spiritual aspects began to influence my perspective, and I found a sense of peace and homecoming in my practice."

Maude bristled. "So you're saying yoga is your religion? I'm a Christian, and that's the same as worshiping a false god, isn't it?"

"No, not at all. I'm saying that when I come to the mat, I can work out all of my problems and brainstorm great ideas. Most importantly, I can connect with myself and even pray. That feeling of connectedness spurred me on to become a yoga teacher so that I could share the benefits with others and, hopefully, give them the tools they need to transform their lives as I did."

As the rest of our coffee hour faded to random anecdotes and silly stories, I pondered Bella's transformation and how much of me I recognized in her story. If yoga had done all that for her in a relatively short period of time, it was worth looking into. I decided to get her new cell number and give her a call to learn more. The need to connect to my inner self was strong; if yoga could help, it deserved a second chance.

Is that why so many seek refuge in yoga? To connect to themselves? I always thought it was just about flexibility; who knew it was so much deeper? Gabby might be right about the therapeutic implications helping with my neuromuscular issues, too.

Later that day, I did a little research. I started with a basic definition. According to the Internet, yoga is a system of exercises practiced to promote control of the body and mind.

Control over the mind and body was an interesting concept. I didn't know if anyone or anything could control my mind; it sort of had a mind of its own. However, I could definitely use some help controlling my body. I had begun to lose mobility in my arms, and my legs were getting weaker again.

There wasn't much to lose by giving yoga another try, except for my pride, but that was long gone anyway. I called Bella. When we met for coffee a few days later, it was just the two of us. She looked as radiant as she had before. There was no mistaking her transformation.

"Bella, I have to tell you how impressed I was by you the other day." She laughed. "Me? Why?"

"Because we both know those women pretty well. That group can be a tough crowd and not the most open. Still, you shared your perspective without hesitation. That was really brave of you."

"Why wouldn't I? Speaking one's truth should never be shameful."

Her words bounced around in my head like one of those little rubber balls. *Why not say what's going on in my mind without worry or shame, because it's my truth?* I honestly had never thought of that. What a profound statement. "I just can't believe you changed this much by joining a yoga class."

"It's a little more involved than that. Yoga is a way of thinking, too. It's a state of being. You push yourself out of your comfort zone in a safe environment. That, in turn, opens you to do the same out in the world. I guess it is all about building self-trust."

I nodded, pretending I knew what she was talking about and then stopped suddenly. "What do you mean exactly?"

"My practice is always evolving. When I'm in a class and try a new pose, I have to trust that my body has the ability to do it. If I don't make it fully into my stance, I can always fall back on the mat and try again. Eventually, if I set my intention to perfect the stance, I will get it. I just need to trust myself and have faith in my body.

Trust and faith go hand in hand, just as strength and flexibility do . . . in yoga and in life. Eventually, each crosses over to the other until they are interchangeable, like the yin/yang symbol."

I thought about my disease. Myasthenia gravis essentially unplugs the nerves from the muscles; they don't trust or talk to each other anymore. My body had been an internal war zone for a long time. I wondered if yoga could help bring peace to both my body and mind.

We are all dealing with something on some level. Some of us experience mental and emotional stress or physical issues, while others are simply searching for deeper meaning. My biggest issue most days was a physical problem with a very long name, but maybe yoga could bring a little peace to all of our problems, no matter the issue.

Interrupting my train of thought, Bella continued. "I often call yoga a practice, but lately I've been approaching it as a conversation. Each day, my body is a little different in strength and flexibility. The same is true for my mind. While I'm on my mat, an intimate dialogue between my body, mind, and soul takes place. Each aspect learns to express itself and listen to the other parts. Sometimes one of the group is really bossy or lazy or sore. Yoga is a safe place where all parties can have their say while the others listen and show compassion. When I am open to myself, I can open up to what God has in store for me, as well."

Her gaze seemed distant as she continued. "When I'm in that sacred space of my practice, I can fully open up my body, releasing the crystallized assumptions of my past experiences and entering a place of possibility."

I wasn't completely clear about what she was saying, but if it had anything to do with the look of total serenity on her face, I was in.

Maybe.

"I want to release the crystallized assumptions of my past experiences and enter a place of possibility, too, whatever that means, but I have some serious physical challenges. I'm not the same person you once knew."

She lovingly ignored the physical changes in my appearance, caused by the many medications that ravaged my skin and seemingly aged me overnight, and the sunglasses I wore nonstop to protect my eyes from sunlight. "What's changed?"

My body slumped in shame as I gazed at the floor. When I replied, my voice was barely audible. "A few years ago, I was practically running marathons before breakfast. The new me is happy when she can manage to brush her teeth in the morning. My breakfast now consists of the truckload of pills I have to take just to do the basic daily tasks. My friends only see me when I am at my best, usually in the morning, when I look and sound semi-normal. I don't show them the other side, the one my family sees. By evening, when I'm tired and worn out physically, my staggering gait makes me look drunk. Sometimes I can't move at all, and my vision is even worse than normal. It's not a pretty sight. There are days that I can't even get out of bed or lift my head from the pillow. Other days, I am fine in the morning or at rest, but if I do something to overexert my body, it just stops working. I have no control over when it occurs. My family knows that when this happens I need to lie down, but I am afraid I will scare other people if they see me that way. I may not look sick, but my body tells a different story."

The silence between us grew unbearable.

Finally, she spoke. "And?"

I sat taller in my chair. "And I guess I'm trying to say that as much as I want the mental side of yoga, I don't know if I can do it physically. I think it may be too hard for me now."

"So? What if it isn't too hard and you can do it? How will you know unless you try? Do you really want to be *that* guy?"

Confused, I asked, "What guy would that be?"

"The guy who sits around all weekend watching football on TV and eating potato chips while talking about the glory days of high school when he was the star quarterback."

"I'm not following."

She casually stroked a dog that had walked over to her. "He lives in the past, focusing on what once was. He doesn't even see who he is now or how he has changed."

I laughed. "Oh, trust me; I see all too clearly how I've changed."

The dog's owner was trying to pull him away to finish their walk. Bella's new canine friend looked at her longingly as if to persuade her to take him home with her.

"Yes, but you only see what you can't do now; you are even embarrassed by it."

"Well, it is embarrassing to fall over when you are in the middle of a conversation with someone." I reached out to pet the pooch but pulled my hand back when the dog gave a warning growl.

"I'm sure it is, but it goes to my original point."

"Which was?"

"It's not about falling over; it's about how you handle getting up. You should come to my chair yoga class. The whole thing is taught to people while they are sitting. Some come because they are elderly and others because they are in a wheelchair or rehabbing. There are all sorts of reasons. What's important isn't the reason they do the poses in a chair but the fact that they are there every week."

I felt a little insulted by her offer. "So you're recommending a handicapped class?"

She rolled her eyes. "I think you might want to think about what that means. I work with a high school student who made his comeback to the soccer field a year and a half after his leg was amputated due to cancer. He played goalie for the junior varsity team and then competed at the varsity level his junior and senior year. Now he is on the American national team for the Paralympics in track and field. Does he consider himself handicapped?"

"No, I guess not."

"Do you believe he spends his days talking about what he used to do before he lost his leg? Or does he accept where he is in this moment and work with what he's got?"

"Probably the latter."

"Exactly. And that is part of what yoga is all about: accepting where you are in your journey and loving yourself and others, not in spite of it but because of it."

"So the only people who are truly handicapped are those who think they are?"

"If we release the mind, the body will follow. That is why we talk about clearing the mind of senseless chatter when we meditate at the end of each practice. Most of what we hear in our minds is fear based anyway. If we can do it on a regular basis, we can bring harmony to the chaos in our heads."

I thought about the chaos in my own head. Even after all my therapy, I still limited my physical boundaries out of fear and shame. Who knew I would turn into one of "those guys" who always looked backward.

She watched me have an entire conversation with myself in my mind. When I finally came out of my mental haze, I noticed her smile. It was really interesting to me, because it was a real smile. She was honestly happy. It was not the fake smile you get when you greet the other moms on the way to school in the morning or the smile you get in the church parking lot as parishioners scurry to their cars to beat the traffic.

It was an honest-to-goodness smile. I hadn't seen one of those in a long time. Nor had I worn one on my own face since . . . I couldn't remember when.

Bella handed me her business card. "Why don't you try one of my basic classes if you don't want to do the chair one? You shouldn't have a problem with the skill level."

"Basic class? Is that for newbies?"

"Sort of. It's an entry level class to get you started. We go a little slower and spend more time focusing on the proper alignment so you don't get hurt."

"I understand all you have said, but I feel that by accepting where I am at this point and not pushing myself to get back to normal, I am submitting to this disease."

She leaned over and put her hand on mine. "Dear friend, you should never submit to anything. Submitting implies that you are giving your power to something or someone else. What I'm suggesting is that you surrender or stop resisting and just go with where you are from this point on. We all have our own ax to grind; it's part of being alive. Some say it's the best part, because it helps us discover who we really are and what we are made of. You don't have to be alone as you travel this road. That's the other thing that is special about the yoga community. The people in my classes learn to forgive themselves when their bodies do not respond the way they want them to, which helps us forgive others, as well. When you learn to trust yourself, you will also learn to trust them. It happens symbiotically. It's a safe way to walk openly in the world and stop hiding from what is. Just as I had to do when I faced financial ruin. As I said, we all have something we are working on."

My emotions were raw, and tears began to stream down my face. I hadn't been very honest with others . . . or myself, for that matter, by showing them only the best of me and not the uglier, weaker, diseased side. I wondered if that is something we all do, even those without an autoimmune issue.

I felt no judgment at all from the woman before me. It made me realize I had been living with judgment my entire life. It hadn't come from my family and friends but from within. How many years had I spent not measuring up to my own expectations? How many of us are doing the same thing to ourselves all day long?

I said, "What was that quote from Eleanor Roosevelt we learned in high school? If I'm remembering right, it was 'No one can make you feel inferior without your consent.' I guess if I fall on my face, literally, I can handle the humiliation. If they don't mind, why should I?"

She laughed. "Eleanor also said, 'A woman is like a tea bag; you never know how strong she is until she gets in hot water.'"

My tears of sadness and regret turned to tears of laughter as we clinked our disposable coffee cups together in unity.

I promised to attend one of her classes someday. She seized the moment, knowing I would probably chicken out once I got home.

"I am teaching a class in about an hour. I have an extra mat in my car. No time better than the present, right?"

CHAPTER 33

WITH NO EXCUSES readily available, I took my first yoga class an hour later. My heart pounded, and I felt like throwing up from anxiety as I sat quietly on a borrowed mat. Until then, I hadn't pushed my body to see what it could really do for fear it would push back. I wanted to explain to the class, which was completely unaware of my issues, that I was way out of my comfort zone and felt incredibly brave for showing up. I also wanted to announce that I had a neuromuscular autoimmune disease, so they would understand if I suddenly fell over. That seemed a bit much to say to a bunch of strangers, so I sat as close to the exit as possible instead and tried to become invisible.

I did invisible pretty well.

We started with a meditation. Mona had encouraged me to meditate, but I could never find the time. In retrospect, I realize that finding the time was more the lesson than the actual meditation. I didn't have much interest in the concept, but it was a great time filler, so I gladly joined in. Besides, since we were lying down during meditation, the odds of falling over were minimal.

The next part of the class wasn't as easy. Bella offered gentle corrections for our yoga positions. She was equally kind to all of us. I noticed that even the "normal" folk in the class were wobbling and grabbing the walls for balance. I was happy to see that we were all struggling together.

Bella had explained the connection between the microcosm of yoga in a classroom and the macrocosm of life, and I was beginning to comprehend her metaphor. She said when we get off kilter during our journey, as we do in yoga, we simply need to accept it and move on to find our equilibrium again.

I progressed in the classes over the next few weeks and noticed that yoga gradually changed my perspective towards my physical form as well as my spiritual outlook.

In my twenties, my body and I had a love/hate relationship . . . probably more hate than love. As many women do, I compared various characteristics, including my size and shape, to those of other women and usually came up short. I would punish my body by over exercising or eating improperly, not connecting the dots that I was actually punishing the rest of my being, as well.

It wore me out.

In my thirties, I became a baby production company, either warehousing and growing new life or feeding it. Although the process was wonderful, there was not much time for self-nurturing.

Sometimes I wonder if not taking care of myself physically and emotionally during adulthood contributed to illness later.

Through yoga, I finally understood that the mind, body, and spirit really are connected. I felt my mind completely relax and listen to my spirit when I was in the yoga poses. It was as if they were finding their way home to each other, the way couples do once they start to reconnect. Yoga opened the channels of communication between all three for the first time since my youth. I started to respect my body for all its strengths and weaknesses, incorporating it into more of a complete me instead of various parts that needed to be improved because they weren't good enough.

I returned to her classes again and again. Some days I was fully present, and my poses were flawed but full of vitality. Other days, I felt tired and listless. During those classes, I would try several of the positions but spent most of the time curled up in child's pose. No one commented or compared; their eyes were usually closed anyway. I accepted whatever my strength could offer in each moment. I learned to honor my being no matter what it did instead of feeling resentment, as if I'd been betrayed.

Historically, gratitude had not been one of the feelings I had towards my form. Mona had helped heal my mind. Yoga and the breath work that comes with it were healing my relationship with the rest of me.

Without this disease, I would never have embarked on my expedition of self-discovery. How profound, I thought, that I had to literally lose the connection to my physical self in order to begin a relationship with all facets of me.

One day after class ended, Bella asked, "How are you doing?"

Before I could form a response, I wondered why I always seemed to wait until something was pried from my hands to make space for new possibilities. Why couldn't I be more open-minded and willing to try different things? Where did the fear come from? Is the unknown really that frightening? I'd learned that when I simply let go, the shift I make is often better than my current state. Of course, it wasn't often that I allowed myself to simply let go. Wouldn't it be better to avoid suffering for growth and instead learn with ease and grace? Maybe that was part of what yoga was all about, more trust and less holding on for dear life.

In the end, all I could say was "I don't know what to think."

She smiled the kind of smile that involves a lot of teeth and a crinkly nose. My kids call it a full-face smile. "Then you got it! You aren't supposed to think at all; you just do. Feel the poses until you become them and they become you."

I wasn't sure we were at that stage of the game, but I was more than willing to fake it till I made it.

She hugged me tight. After she let go, she said, "You are never a victim to your life but the creator of it. It may not look the way you envisioned, but it will be exactly what you need in order to learn the lessons that were intended for you."

For some reason, my mind flashed to the patients at my oncologist's office and the sense of peace they seemed to possess in the face of uncertainty. I was just as uncertain every day I lived with my own diagnoses but now felt that same peace in my being, as well, with an added bonus of self-contentment. I was learning to surrender my challenges, no longer resisting my body when I thought it had failed, which allowed me to focus more on the strengths I still had. Letting go of what I couldn't control freed me to develop other potential gifts I never knew existed. I'm not sure that would have happened if I had remained an average mom with no physical issues.

I thanked Bella for the new perspective yoga had offered and asked if there was anything else she thought I should investigate to further my travels.

She looked over my shoulder.

"Hey, Pamela, do you have a minute?"

I turned to see a beautiful woman with long, curly brown hair. As she walked toward us, I noticed that she was small in stature but big in energy. "Sure. What's up?"

"This is my friend, Lisa. She really needs your help."

I turned to Bella. "I do?"

"You do. Pamela does nutrition work. One of the things she can help you with is your diet."

I felt almost insulted. After giving birth to three children, I could still fit into my wedding dress. Part of that was due to my intermittent inability to chew, but no one needed to know that. "What's wrong with my diet? My weight is just fine, according to the scale!"

Pamela rolled her eyes. "I wish I had a dollar for every person who thought the scale had anything to do with nutrition. If you have any type of health issues, what you put into your body is even more important."

Did she know I was sick? "What do you mean?"

As if Bella had read my mind, she interrupted. "Pamela specializes in cleaning up the diets of clients who have had various illnesses."

Pamela explained. "Some people choose not to do traditional Western medicine but instead control their medical issues with diet . . . depending on the issues, of course. You would be surprised how high our success rate is for things like type 2 diabetes, irritable bowel syndrome, celiac disease, ulcers, you name it. We have even had some luck in assisting with the healing process of cancer patients."

My skepticism may have bled into my tone. "Really? If you can cure cancer just by eating oranges or whatever, where do I sign up?"

Pamela had a presence about her I hadn't seen before. It was almost as if she were glowing from the inside out. She reached into her bag and produced a business card. "It's not quite that easy, but give me a call when you are ready and we can set something up."

After I left the yoga studio, I got into my car and surveyed its contents. In the passenger seat was the half-eaten muffin I'd called breakfast. Candy wrappers from my son and his friends covered the floor, and there was a spare granola bar in the glove compartment for emergencies.

Not my finest hour when it came to feeding myself or my family.

Maybe I could learn something from Pamela. I thought the foods my family ate were relatively healthy, but I suppose if they were, I wouldn't be so relatively unhealthy.

I hadn't considered the potential correlation between what I ingested and the breakdown of my body before. What was it they say? You are what you eat?

Seeing all the different angles of a situation always makes me think about the multitude of elements that can contribute to a problem. It also promises hope that there are just as many possibilities for a cure.

CHAPTER 34

Write your goals in concrete and your plans in sand.
Anonymous

THE NEXT MORNING, I stood naked in front of my bathroom mirror before hopping into the shower. I was a woman in her forties trying to come to terms with the physical effects of previous cancers and an autoimmune disease, along with the normal processes of aging.

I studied myself with an almost scientific eye, not sure what to think of the battered body that stood before me or how to have empathy for the vessel I live in. I sensed it was finally time to let go of self-judgment, but that is sometimes easier said than done. The judger living in my head is a pretty powerful guy.

As I contemplated the reflection of the scarred, weak figure in the mirror, my mind displayed another vision. I saw a warrior returning from battle. Although weary and war torn, she knows that ultimately she has won her quest, because whatever happens to her on the outside can't damage the soul she has successfully protected deep within her. She understands that her body is the shield guarding her spirit from destruction. No matter how damaged she looks on the surface, her heart remains beautiful.

While the heat rose from the shower and the room filled with steam, I came back to the present to view my body through different eyes. It was the same broken-down vehicle that seemed to stall at every intersection, but instead of seeing myself with the critical eye that only looks with disdain, I looked with compassion. My body might not be perfect, but it has carried me through both good and rough times and enabled me to learn invaluable lessons I would never have known had life been different.

Saying a little prayer of gratitude, I vowed to no longer be filled with regret every time I thought about what I could no longer do. Instead, I would try to focus on all that was possible. For a change, I decided that I would give myself the same understanding I seem to show everyone else.

CHAPTER 35

Let food be thy medicine and medicine be thy food.
Hippocrates

PAMELA AND I MET a few days later. Before she arrived, I'd quickly emptied the cabinets of all the cereal, cookies, brownies, potato chips, and anything else she would probably shun. For the first time ever, my kids fought over who would take out the trash. They stood beside the house with the bag for quite a while. I still don't know how much of it actually made it to the can.

Shaking my head in disgust while secretly wishing I had eaten the last Snickers myself made me realize that changing my family's eating habits wouldn't be as easy as I'd hoped.

I started to think about when I was a child. My mother and I didn't have much money, so we ate a lot of Hamburger Helper and those TV dinners with the little compartments for each portion. If I'd been a really good girl, I would get the kind with the chocolate pudding in the middle for dessert. I loved the chocolate pudding. Still do. Back then, frozen dinners were considered a balanced meal, because they included green beans in one section and meatloaf in another, not that I ate anything but the mashed potatoes and the pudding.

In my mind, I was doing loads better feeding my own family. But, then, I was great at comparing the things I did to something worse so I would come out looking better.

After inspecting my cabinets, I wondered how much better off we really were with a diet involving so much processed and sweetened food. At that moment, I was glad to be alone in my sugar shame. Seriously, who was I trying to kid? We definitely had room for improvement in the nutrition department.

After she sat down, I offered Pamela some green tea and a piece of fruit; it was the healthiest food in the house and all I could come up with on such short notice.

I was curious how she came to her type of work. "I hope you don't mind my asking, but it seems that people in complementary fields of medicine often come to them because they or someone they love has been sick before. How did you get into the nutrition business?"

She looked out the window as she talked. "We are from the South. Our diets were filled with fried foods for dinner, biscuits and gravy for breakfast, and sandwiches slathered with mayonnaise for lunch. No church function was complete without a multitude of baked goods. I watched as my family and friends grew to alarming sizes. They didn't see the harm in it, because our entire society was getting fat, as well. Then my father started taking statins, enzyme inhibitors to lower his high cholesterol. Blood pressure medications followed. The doctor mentioned casually that he might want to lose some weight. Unfortunately, he didn't give my dad any information as to why or how to do it effectively, so my father just ignored the half-hearted advice. He died from a heart attack when he was sixty years old and more than 150 pounds overweight.

My mother and a brother were also taking medication for their cholesterol and blood pressure. One day, I saw them wash down their pills with a coke after eating fried chicken and French fries for lunch, and a light bulb went off in my head. We were all slowly killing ourselves with the good old American diet, and someone had to say something. I decided to be the voice of reason for the safety of my family and myself. I felt that it was up to me to educate as many people as would listen so that we could live longer, happier, healthier lives."

"Did it work?" I regretted asking the question the moment it came out of my mouth.

She looked down and started playing with her hands. "After my father passed away, my brother had his own heart attack. He lived, but at forty years old, he was still very overweight and eventually had a stroke. After that, people started paying attention."

I felt her pain. "It is too bad something tragic has to happen to inspire people."

Her smile looked a bit wistful. "I agree, but because of it my mother and brother each lost more than one hundred pounds, and the rest of the family started exercising and eating a more balanced diet. They still ate their chicken and gravy, but at least it was the exception rather than the rule in their diet. My dad would be happy to know he didn't die in vain. And it inspired me to work with people who have chronic illnesses such as diabetes, autoimmune disease, gout, and cancer, along with anyone else who wants to improve their quality of life."

"You seriously think you can cure cancer with food?" I'll admit there was a hint of sarcasm in my tone.

She sat up straighter in her chair as if defending her stance. "Well, smarty pants, some do believe they can cure some cancers with diet. However, I try to help those going through radiation, chemo, or any other medical treatments keep their nutrition up so they can feel as good as possible. As you know, when you don't feel well, you tend to get sloppy with good eating habits. Also, when you are too tired or weak to eat, you either grab something easy or don't eat at all. Neither is healthy. There are lots of things to keep on hand that aren't junk and can help you have more energy and feel better."

That certainly made sense. It reminded me of when I was going through chemo and radiation. Food tasted terrible to me, even when I was hungry, which wasn't very often. Looking back at all the empty calories I ate made me wish I had packed them with real nutrition to make me feel stronger at the time.

It also made me think about how many years I had lived on empty calories. When our bodies are filled with nothing but fluff, we become nothing better than fluff. Life has such a deeper meaning when I choose to look at it with more purpose. I was grateful for the richness I felt through fuller, more meaningful experiences.

I wondered if Pamela practiced what she preached, though. Casually, I asked, "How do *you* eat?"

"I'm a vegan, and so are a few my family members now."

Like many of us who don't fully understand veganism, I automatically made a sour face as I thought of how unappealing that sounded. I knew a few vegans, and they were the most obnoxious people around. They picked around in their food at restaurants and asked the poor servers how everything on their plate was prepared. I'd also seen them protesting outside fast-food places like Kentucky Fried Chicken. I shook off the image of signs with pictures of mangled chickens and brought my focus back to our conversation. "Isn't that kind of extreme?"

"My family thought so when I first approached them with the idea, but if you consider a plant-based diet versus my brother's triple bypass surgery and the lifelong supply of medications many of my cousins have to buy . . . well, which is more extreme?"

When she put it that way, the decision seemed like a no brainer. Although, sadly, I know many people who would prefer to stay on their meds and shop in the chubby section of the store rather than give up their double cheeseburgers. The only thing I understood about the term *vegan* was that you don't eat anything that comes from an animal. Unfortunately, all I could picture were those crazy people who wear multiple layers of ill-fitting clothing with frumpy shoes and attend rallies to free the whales or something.

Not that there is anything wrong with vegans. They just seem to be a little more opinionated than everyone else.

Or maybe just louder.

Of course, it could be that I'm the opinionated one, holding a preconceived idea about vegans. I decided to keep all my thoughts to myself for the time being and just listen to what she had to say.

I liked talking about other people's eating habits but wasn't completely clear how it could help me with a neurological autoimmune issue.

Looking at the bowl of slightly fuzzy fruit on my counter, I asked, "Do you really think you can help me?"

She smiled and pulled some books from the bag she'd brought with her. "Mountains of research have been done all over the world that discuss the connection between nutrition and overall wellness, especially when our health is compromised. Think about it; how could it not? When we put bad gas in a car, we get a clogged-up engine. The same holds true for bad food. We need to clean our engines and add the proper fuel to get them to run at maximum efficiency."

"But my problem is neurological." I understood the connection between food and the digestive system, but the nerves?

"Well, did you know that omega-3 supplements and certain fats help coat the nerve endings?"

"Uh, no."

"They are also great for reducing eye dryness. Didn't you say that was a facet of your disease? And that is just for starters. There are lots of ways we can give your body the best chance it has to heal by feeding it the right nutrients. Why not be a participant in your healing process? This is one of the best and easiest ways to do it."

My goal has always been to be part of the process and the solution. I wanted to heal from the inside out. What better way to do it than with food? I had a feeling it sounded easier than it would actually be, but I decided to give it a try by investigating further.

"Where do I begin?"

She laughed. "I always say, 'We start with today because that is all we have.' How do you think you have been doing in this area of your life?"

She had no idea what she was getting into.

"I was doing pretty well, at least I thought I was, but then I got sick and lost the ability to chew or swallow anything that didn't come out of a straw. I went without solid food for well over a year."

She didn't look as alarmed as I thought she would. Usually, when I tell people that, they look at me with horror and a little pity, too.

"So what did you do when that happened?"

"I learned to juice. I bought one of those super-sized juicers and stuck as many fruits and vegetables in it as I could find. I learned to juice just about anything. I think at one point I accidentally juiced part of my toaster."

She did a double take. "Really?"

Okay. Maybe we didn't have the same sense of humor. But, then, my daughter says nobody gets me anyway; she could be right.

"No, but it felt like it. I learned more about juicing than I ever wanted to know. Fortunately, I got stronger, and I can eat some soft foods now."

"Why do you think you got stronger?"

I pondered this question for a minute. "I don't really know why. Little by little, I just did."

She shook her head. "You didn't know it, but your body actually did you a little favor. You had a whole lifetime of toxicity floating around in your system that you cleaned out with all that juice. I'm sure it was a challenging time for you, but your organs probably really appreciated it more than you know. And, just possibly, that is the reason you got stronger, too!"

I had never thought of it that way. I had done a total body cleanse without realizing it.

She put back a few of the books she'd pulled out. "I was going to give you some information about the benefits of juice cleansing, but you already skipped ahead a few steps, so it isn't necessary. Your body is a clean slate now. That is a great place to be, but I'm sure you are now lacking a few nutrients that we need to replace."

She set the rest of the books on the table. "I want you to look these over and see which ones resonate with you. There are lots of ways we can do this, but I find that unless a diet resonates with a person, she won't stay in the game."

"What do you mean?"

She pulled a book out of the pile. "This is the Atkins diet book. I absolutely hate this book and everything it recommends, but men typically love the eating plan."

I looked at her, puzzled. "If you don't like it, why have it in your mix?"

"Because if you follow it exactly, you will lose weight, and a healthy weight is better than being obese. My hope is that once the process starts, the person will become more aware of what he is putting into his body. The more aware we become and the better we feel about ourselves, the faster unhealthy habits change. It gets the ball rolling."

"So thin with lots of bad food is better than fat and lots of bad food?"

"Sort of. The food isn't exactly bad. There are just much healthier ways of eating. But as I said, once someone starts losing weight and exercising, she becomes more conscious of what goes into her mouth. That's when we introduce even more nutritious foods and healthful ways of eating. My goal is to help people understand that they don't need a diet; it's a lifestyle change that will help them accomplish their long-term goals of health and fitness. But that is only an example. You have to find what works for you. There are many different theories, and they tend to contradict each other, which can get a little confusing. You have to go with the one that works best for your body and situation."

Looking over the mound of books, I suddenly got overwhelmed. "So where do I begin?"

"The first thing I have my clients do is a cleanse. Since you are already cleansed after all the juicing you have been doing, we can move to the next step. Read some of these, and let's talk again in a few days. And I strongly recommend watching the movie "Forks Over Knives." It will change your life. At least it did mine, and it's done the same thing for many others. Did you know that the American diet is creating a generation in which the children of today will likely live shorter lives than their parents?"

I looked around at my kitchen. "Because of their diet?"

"Yep. We are creating a society that has lost its way and forgotten how to eat. It is literally killing us. It is time to wake up."

My eyes were wide open to the concept. Painful as it might be for me and my people at home, I knew it was the right direction to go for all of us. I wanted to give everyone the best chance I could for a healthy life.

After she left, I tossed all the reading material onto my bed to sift through it. I wasn't sure where we were going or if such a severe change was even something I could do with my family, but I really wanted to try to better fortify our bodies.

She was right. We spend much of our lives unconsciously eating whatever is convenient or tasty, never thinking about its contents. Imagine what would happen if we looked a little closer at what we are putting in our mouths. Once we realize what all that fat, sugar, and salt is doing to our insides, I wonder if we would ever eat another donut or candy bar again.

I thought about my children again and what they were learning about food. Food is fun. Food is love. Food is a way to connect with friends. Food is just about everything except a way to nurture and heal one's body. How did we miss that in the education department? Maybe some of us got the real message, but I certainly didn't. For me, food was comfort. During and after college, I made brownies when I was sad, cookies when I was anxious, and pasta or another heavy carb when I was cold and lonely. Thinking about the nutritional content as the fork passed my lips never hit my radar.

I recently watched a documentary about the hot lunch program at elementary schools in France (don't ask) and I found it fascinating. Every morning, a chef visits the local market and buys food to prepare fresh, locally harvested meals. She said it was important for children to understand where their food originated and how it affects their bodies. None of what the French schools served was white, processed, or microwaved, and the cost was about the same as what we spend in the states. Who dictates our school food programs? Swanson? Pillsbury?

Most of my education about food came from TV commercials and ads while I was growing up. Eat this, and you will feel better. It worked until the self-loathing for adding unwanted calories to my list of issues kicked in.

What we feed our bodies isn't just a food issue; it is a love issue. When we feed our bodies with healthy, vitamin-and-mineral-dense food, we are feeding our souls, too. We are telling are bodies that they are important, and we want to take care of them and love them for sustaining us through life. How many of us love and accept ourselves enough to consciously eat with gratitude? My guess is that there aren't many. Yes, I am staring at the floor in shame, as well.

My guess is that most of us accept the lies we hear about food and go about our days asleep at the wheel, as I have done. Maybe it is time to wake up and love ourselves enough to pay attention to what is happening at our kitchen table, for our sakes and for our children's health.

CHAPTER 36

The whiter the bread, the faster you're dead.
Daniel Amen

AFTER THE KIDS WERE ASLEEP and the house was finally quiet, I returned to the mound of books on my bed. The first one I picked up focused on cleansing. Even though I was "clean," my family wasn't, so I started reading. The book explained that there are as many options for juice cleanses as there are fruits and vegetables in season. The author described juice fasting as a great way to kick start and restore our digestive system and lose weight at the same time. Also, when we are dehydrated, the body may feel hunger when we really need fluids. He said juice is a perfect way to rehydrate.

The book offered sample recipes for beginning the process of cleansing the body and clearing the mind. As I read, I imagined the looks on the faces of my family members as I served them each recipe.

Vegetable Super Juice
1 whole cucumber
4 sticks celery
2-4 handfuls spinach
8 lettuce leaves
Optional boosters: parsley and fresh alfalfa sprouts
Water

My son might claim child abuse due to forced starvation if I offered him that one. I continued to read.

Healing Juice
3-4 carrots
125g fresh spinach
Handful of flat-leaf parsley
2-3 stalks celery
Water

That recipe would be less green and not as strong, so it was a possibility. But I continued my search.

Blood Builder (iron-enriched)
2 bunches grapes
6 oranges
8 lemons, peeled
1/4 cup honey
Water

We were getting warmer. At least it sounded sweet. Every child I know loves food that is sweet, even if it is healthy.

Pina Colada
Half a cup each coconut water and coconut milk
1 teaspoon vanilla
2-3 cups fresh or frozen pineapple
Ice

The winner! It was sweet and healthy and reminded me of our trip to Hawaii, a perfect way of easing my family into the juice concept.

An endless array of options would enable me to mix it up a little. I knew from my previous experience with juicing that it was simple enough to throw the ingredients in a blender or juicer, add water and ice if desired, and drink. And with so many different fruits and vegetables available year round in California, my family would benefit from a variety of vitamins without popping supplements, and it would be less expensive. God knows we spent enough on medications and vitamins already.

After putting the juice book in the keep pile, I flipped through another one that talked about something called phytonutrients. The author explained that these plant-derived nutrients sustain human life by helping the immune system fight inflammatory responses and infections. That seemed right up my alley, so I held onto it, as well.

The third book described the way refined sugar and processed foods break down the body's tissues. Hours passed as I reviewed literature discussing fad diets, celebrity diets, the diet of monks in Asia, and everything in between. I read until I was so confused that all I really wanted to do was eat a brownie.

Brownies always made everything better.

Maybe not. I had learned too much about the evils of sugar, and Lord knows what else those little brown nuggets of goodness contained that could probably kill me.

After all that research, I thought it would be easier to throw the baby out with the bathwater and give up on the whole nutrition concept rather than figuring out what would work best for us. It was frustrating to see so many books fight over the right way to eat.

Who do I believe? Maybe I really should forget the whole idea.

Blocking that idea from my mind, I pressed on.

But first I went to the kitchen for a brownie, sugar be damned.

After reading until my eyes felt like they were going to fall out, one thing became glaringly clear: there is a lot of data that claims to support any and every kind of food plan. Well, maybe it's not research in a strict sense, but there certainly is a lot of information out there. I decided to put all the books away and give Pamela a call in the morning.

*   *   *

Unsure where to begin with so many questions swirling around in my mind, I started with the obvious. "So, Pamela, I read the books you gave me and did some research of my own on the Internet and decided that the food business is very confusing."

She didn't sound surprised. "How did you feel when you were reading? Did anything strike you?"

"What do you mean?"

"Once our awareness is tuned in, most of us will have an "aha" moment when it comes to nutrition. All we have to do is find the door to our truth."

Was she a nutritionist or a therapist?

It seems that no matter where I turn, I am being guided to my truth in every aspect of my life, whatever that means. I suspect that at some point I unconsciously set truth as my soul's intention, kind of like a secret contract my spirit wrote so I could find my way.

One of these days, I hope to find the compass to my roadmap so I know which direction I am headed.

I continued. "The truth is that I don't know what to believe."

My statement didn't apply only to my diet, but I wasn't ready to discuss the other aspects. We were just getting to know each other, after all.

She was very patient with me. "I have an idea. Why don't you research diets for the prevention of cancer or autoimmune diseases and see what you come up with. That may speak to you a little more clearly and set you on your way."

"Okay, but don't most dieticians just hand clients a list of foods to eat and those to avoid and send you packing?"

She laughed. "Some do, but I'm not one of them. And guess how many of those clients follow the plan or are compliant anyway?"

"Not many?"

"No, not many at all. If you aren't invested in something as important as what to feed your body, then you typically won't be invested in anything else regarding your health. It's not just about what you eat; it's about becoming conscious of how you eat and how that relates to the rest of your world, as well. We have become a society that isn't paying attention, asleep at the wheel. It is time to wake up to what we are doing to ourselves and our world. What better way than to start at the beginning: how we eat."

I was starting to understand what she was trying to convey. "Are you saying that once we become mindful of the decisions we make about how we take care of our bodies, we become more aware of other health-related choices, too?"

"That is exactly what I am saying. We also get the chance to consciously listen to our bodies and, hopefully, respond accordingly.

You have no idea how many clients tell me they are highly allergic to dairy but eat ice cream anyway, because they 'can't help themselves.' The more attention and respect we pay to our systems, the better we feel."

I thought about what she'd said. She was right. Thanks to the pace of our lives and the steady stream of electronics and multitasking, we really are disconnecting from ourselves and the needs of our bodies. It reminded me of a woman I'd seen driving on the freeway while eating a burger and talking on the phone. There was a lot going on there with no real consciousness of any of it, especially what she was putting in her body.

She also almost ran us off the road.

When I Googled diets for cancer prevention, I quickly discovered numerous ideas. For instance, multiple articles stated that focusing on plant-based food is better if you are sick, because plants have less fat and more fiber, along with an arsenal of cancer-fighting nutrients. It said that these three elements work together to support the immune system and help your body fight off disease. This includes a variety of vegetables, fruits, and whole grains. A plant-based diet means eating mostly foods that come from plants: vegetables, fruits, nuts, grains, and beans.

Also, the less a food is processed—meaning the less it's been cooked, peeled, stripped of nutrients, or otherwise altered from the way it came out of the ground—the more nutrient rich that food will be.

In addition, I learned that different types of fruits and vegetables are more effective than others in preventing various types of cancers. According to multiple websites, a link has been seen between the consumption of certain foods and a reduction in the incidence of specific cancers. For example, onions protect against stomach cancer; tomatoes may prevent prostate cancer; garlic reduces the likelihood of colon cancer; and eating fruit can lower the incidence of cancer in the mouth, throat, lung, and stomach.

Several sites recommended simplifying your diet and aiming for a minimum of five servings of a variety of vegetables and fruits every day. They suggest eating unprocessed grains (whole wheat, oats, barley, bulgur, quinoa, and brown rice) or legumes (beans and lentils) at every meal and avoiding refined starches like sugar, white bread, and cereals not made with whole grains.

Andrew Weil, MD, a noted expert on integrated health, mentioned in an article that chronic inflammation is often the root cause of many serious illnesses, including heart disease, several cancers, and Alzheimer's disease. We've all seen inflammation on the surface of the body, which appears as local redness, heat, swelling, and pain. He explained that it's the cornerstone of the body's healing response, bringing more nourishment and more immune activity to a site of injury or infection. But when inflammation persists or serves no purpose, it damages the body and causes illness. Stress, lack of exercise, genetic predisposition, and exposure to toxins like secondhand tobacco smoke can all contribute to such chronic inflammation, but dietary choices play a big role, as well. He said that learning how specific foods influence the inflammatory process is the best strategy for containing it and reducing long-term disease risks.

His anti-inflammatory diet is not a diet in the popular sense but a way of selecting and preparing foods based on scientific knowledge of how they can help your body maintain optimum health. Along with influencing inflammation, this diet claims to provide steady energy and ample vitamins, minerals, essential fatty acids, dietary fiber, and protective phytonutrients.

Countless websites pointed in the same direction: meat, dairy, and processed foods are no friends to the sick or those who want optimum health. I went back to my books and pulled out *The China Study*, written by respected nutrition and health researcher Dr. T. Colin Campbell, who was raised on a dairy farm.

Early in his career as a researcher, Dr. Campbell believed that better health came from eating more meat, milk, and eggs. On a project in the Philippines, he worked with malnourished children to find out why so many were diagnosed with liver cancer, typically an adult disease. He found that those who ate the highest protein diets were the ones most likely to get liver cancer. He reviewed other reports from around the world that agreed with the findings of his research. This project discovered more than eight thousand statistical correlations between various dietary factors and disease.

Dr. Campbell concluded that "people who ate the most animal-based foods got the most chronic disease. Those who ate the most plant-based foods were the healthiest and tended to avoid chronic disease."

I also read a book called *The Autoimmune Epidemic*, which reported that the number of people in the United States who succumb to autoimmune diseases is skyrocketing. It made me wonder how much nutrition was involved in breaking down the immune response, as well.

Nutrition cannot be taken lightly by those with compromised health. Even our own medical establishment is finally coming around to this conclusion. That was the aha moment Pamela promised I would have.

I had an appointment to meet with her in the morning, and I knew what I needed to do. However, I didn't know how or where to start.

But that had never stopped me in the past. I guess blind faith in the process is better than no faith at all.

CHAPTER 37

Start where you are. Use what you have. Do what you can.
Arthur Ashe

I WALKED INTO PAMELA'S office and gently dropped my bag of books on her desk.

She looked at them and then at me. "So are you blind after reading all of these?"

Trying to organize my thoughts, I pulled out a notebook filled with questions and comments from my reading. "Well, my vision may be a little blurrier than normal, but I am clear now that anyone with a chronic illness—or any disease, for that matter—should take nutrition seriously. Also, I'm ready for a more plant-based diet. How do I do that?"

She shrugged. "How do you want to do it?"

I glanced at my notes. "I want to be more vegan or vegetarian or maybe both. I guess I'm unclear about the differences."

"That's a good place to start. If you are a vegetarian, you don't consume any animals. What did Phoebe say on the show *Friends*? I think it was 'I eat nothing with a face.' A vegan cuts out animal products, including dairy and eggs."

I could handle not eating anything with a face, but no eggs or dairy sounded a bit extreme. "It would be hard to obtain the right amount of calcium and protein without dairy or eggs, right?"

"Not really. You can get enough calcium by drinking fortified soy, almond, or rice milk and eating almonds and green, leafy vegetables. Milk—actually, most dairy—can be highly inflammatory to the body. And eggs may be one of the unhealthiest food choices due to possible salmonella contamination and artery-clogging cholesterol. Did you know that one egg contains as much cholesterol as three servings of beef?"

"But I've heard that you have to take a large quantity of vitamin supplements if you are vegetarian."

"As long as you are eating a variety of nutrient-dense foods, you would have a higher vitamin content coursing through your blood than most people. Non-meat foods can replace animal protein. Besides, the protein in meat is long chain and second hand. It's like chewing already-chewed gum. You're eating something that has eaten another creature. The fat from the first critter goes directly into the system of the second one. Fat is where all the toxins are stored. Those pollutants end up in your own body fat. And don't even get me started about the stuff we find in the fillers and additives included in ground and other processed meat."

I felt nauseous. "Gross. Go on."

"On the other hand, the amino acids in fresh, organic greens are pure, light-filled, chlorophyll rich, and fresh from the sun and soil. They are ready to be woven into proteins specifically for your body. Greens are my meat of choice."

My nose scrunched up involuntarily. "But digging into a nice, juicy bunch of kale just doesn't sound very appetizing."

"There are ways to make them taste delicious and many different types of greens to choose from. Besides, if top athletes can eat them and pull out peak performances, the rest of us can certainly add greens to our eating plan and stay healthy."

"Which athletes don't use meat as their protein source? I thought it was a big deal to be on a high-protein diet when you are training."

She reached into her desk drawer. "I came across an article that mentions a few super athletes who stick to a strict vegan or vegetarian regime. Here's a track-and-field star who set multiple world records and won two Olympic gold medals while fueled by a purely vegetarian diet. Two of the highest-winning female tennis champs were both committed vegetarians for most of their lives. One of the greatest NBA players in the history of the game is famous for his vegetarianism, evidence that even a huge, athletic individual doesn't need meat to power the body. A certain heavyweight boxer committed to a fully vegan regime. It seems to have done wonders for the prize-winning fighter, as he's slimmer and says he's happier now than he has been in years.

Super Bowl champion Joe Namath said when commenting on his own eating habits, "It shows you don't need meat to play football." Also, a top leader in ultra-marathoning, which involves running anywhere from thirty to one hundred miles at a time, is a lifelong vegan."

Noticing the list was a few pages long and not wanting to miss my next birthday, I put my hand up to stop her. "Okay. Okay. You want to jump to your point?"

"My point is that if athletes like these can do astounding things while making plant-based food choices, mere mortals like us can certainly handle it. The Mexican Tarahumara Indians are considered super athletes. Their diet consists almost entirely of beans, corn, squash, pumpkins, root vegetables, and wild plants and fruits. Their endurance is amazing, as they regularly run up to 120 miles in one day. I can keep going if you want."

Pamela could definitely express her opinion.

"I get it, but I am still concerned about the protein part. My doctor is pushing that pretty hard. He also says I am anemic. How do vegetarians keep their iron levels up?"

"Nuts, beans and rice, soy products such as tofu, dark greens, whey products like seitan, or vegan cheeses. An abundance of non-meat sources of protein and iron are readily available. Ethnic foods regularly include vegan and vegetarian options that are loaded with enough protein to keep your levels up. Plant-based foods are a staple in many other countries."

"I do feel better when I skip heavy, processed foods, but aren't organic items harder to buy and more expensive to cook?"

She pulled out a few cookbooks and handed them to me. "I'll give you some homework. Take these home and try some of the recipes. Pick out a few that are easy to make and that you think the kids would like. Let me know your thoughts when I see you again. Anything can look good on paper, but if it doesn't work on the dinner table, why bother, right?"

Her suggestion seemed practical enough. After I got home that afternoon, I pulled out a couple of the books and flipped straight to the dessert section. It's my favorite part of any cookbook. Some of the recipes seemed pretty basic, with ingredients I already had in my kitchen, so I decided to give them a try. Later that evening, as the children were watching TV, I slid a plate of vegan brownies and peanut butter cookies onto the coffee table.

My son became concerned. I never make dessert midweek. "Mom, are you all right?"

I smiled. "Yes. I'm trying out a new cookbook. Taste these and tell me what you think."

He looked at the plate suspiciously. "Why?"

"What do you mean, why? Can't a mom make dessert once in a while without an interrogation?"

Confused, he said, "No."

My experiment wasn't working out as I'd hoped. "Will you just try the stupid things and tell me if you like them or not? I'm not asking for much here."

Slowly, they approached the plate as if waiting for some phantom booby traps to trigger. When none did, each picked up a brownie and smelled it.

Throwing my hands up in the air, I said, "Oh, for the love of God, people! Just eat them!"

Almost in unison, they shoved them into their mouths. Their expressions slowly changed from worry to delight.

They sampled the cookies next. After a few commercial breaks, the plate was empty.

"So, what do you think?"

They looked at me and smiled. My son was the first to speak. "Not bad, Mom."

Coming from someone who loves his sweets, that was the ultimate compliment. I didn't plan to tell them the treats were made without flour, eggs, or refined sugar. The secret ingredient that I would surely never mention was chickpeas. Who knew beans were a staple ingredient for cookies in the vegan world?

"Thanks, guys. Tomorrow, let's try tofu."

They responded in complete harmony. "No!"

It appeared I would have to ease into that one.

CHAPTER 38

AS I ENTERED PAMELA'S office for my next appointment, I felt the weight of the now chocolate-stained cookbooks stuffed in my bag.

"So, how'd it go?"

Smiling and satisfied, I said, "Great! And not so great."

"What do you mean?"

I took the books out of my bag and set them on her desk. Then I tried to explain. "My brood loved almost everything I made. They liked it enough to entertain the idea of going vegan once in a while. I ended up working meatless meals into our dinner schedule four days last week, and they didn't even notice. I think I am ready to toss out anything that once had a pulse."

"Great! What's the not-so-great part?"

I took a seat in her uncomfortable guest chair. "After thinking through everything we have been talking about, I am now aware that I've been poisoning my family with the over-processed crap we've been eating and want to change everything about our diet."

As we talked, she organized the books she'd loaned me, sorting them according to some mysterious system. "That sounds pretty great, as well, although you may want to do it slowly to avoid freaking anyone out. So what's the not-so-great part?"

"I got a call from my daughter Jordan's teacher. She reminded me that I had signed up to supply snacks for Back to School night. It was a better option than being in charge of their pet lizard during spring break."

"Still not following."

"I thought it would be good to start practicing what I will be preaching to my family and offered to take a veggie tray with some hummus. There was nothing but silence on the other end of the phone. Then I proposed the banana oatmeal cookies the kids found tasty. I could almost hear crickets chirping in the stillness. She was less than interested."

She chuckled. "What did you end up making?"

Practically under my breath, I said, "Chocolate cupcakes with chocolate icing and sprinkles."

"Vegan?"

"Duncan Hines."

"Nice."

"Have you ever tried to talk about nutrition in the public school system? I once told the district nutritionist that I thought serving ice cream as a free snack at 10:00 in the morning was not sending the right message to my kindergartener. Sounding annoyed, she said I was misinformed and assured me it was fine to give them any type of dairy in the morning. When I protested about the sugar content, she said if I was going to be difficult, I needed to take it up with the board and not to bother her again."

"Wow. So what did you do?"

"I told the school that my daughter was allergic to dairy and to stop giving it to her. You have to pick your battles when navigating through twelve years of education times three children. At that particular school, sprinkles are considered a food group and a good one, at that."

She laughed. "I never said it would be easy, especially when there are outside forces involved. Baby steps, right?"

"Baby steps. Even when they are for my babies. Can we move on, or are you giving up on me?"

She turned my way as she put the last book back on its shelf. "Moms are moms first and activists second. We do what we can within the framework we have and hope for the best. That's all we can ask for. I'm far from giving up on you. Let's move on."

Trying another chair, which proved to be equally uncomfortable, I wondered if all health practitioners do that on purpose so you don't stay too long.

I contemplated something she'd said earlier. "Do you honestly think it will ever be possible for us to become a meatless society?"

"I suppose anything can happen. Did you know that in the United States nearly two thousand pounds of grain are consumed per person per year either directly or through food for livestock? People in the rest of the world average about four hundred pounds of grain per year."

"So is that why we are so fat? Or so sick?"

"Not necessarily, but it does help explain why much of the earth's population is starving."

I wasn't seeing the correlation. "Explain, please."

"We are feeding to cows the food that could save human lives. If we ate less meat, as little as 10 percent less per year, we could feed sixty million more people."

"Holy cow. No pun intended."

She laughed again. She was serious about nutrition, but at least she was starting to understand my humor.

She returned to her explanation. "A book titled *Diet for a Small Planet* says that Americans make up about 7 percent of the world's population but consume more than 30 percent of the world's animal foods. The author contends that producing meat to supply humans with protein is grossly inefficient. He claims that the vast expanse of land being used for raising livestock could feed up to twenty times more people if it were planted with crops instead."

"Okay. I get it. But I can't guarantee my teenagers will. Weaning them off burgers and fries will be a painful process."

"The first guideline is to avoid turning diet into another stressor in our lives. Ease into it. People can get crazy about their beliefs, no matter what they choose to eat. I have a friend who feeds her family huge quantities of meat, eggs, butter, and whole milk. I think it's called the GAPS diet. She is militant about their meals and how they are prepared. If you make mealtime a big thing, you and your family end up stressed, which is counterproductive for everyone. It may also cause food rebellion. Mealtimes should be easy and enjoyable. Start small instead of turning your family's world upside down by throwing out all the cookies and putting the bacon on lockdown."

Working with her philosophy on food sounded easier than anticipated. I only wish I'd talked to her before ousting the snacks; I really missed my animal crackers. "How do we start small, then?"

She handed me a brochure picturing a cow with a circle around it and an X through the middle. "Public health schools such as Johns Hopkins and Columbia have designed a campaign called Meatless Monday to help people do just that. Their goal is to help Americans avoid our top four killers . . . heart disease, stroke, diabetes, and cancer . . . by eating meat-free at least one day a week. The program provides recipes, meal plans, nutritional guidelines, cooking tips, and all sorts of other information. It's already being adopted in some schools and hospitals."

Furiously scribbling notes, I thought out loud. "I think my family could handle one meatless day a week on a consistent basis. At least my daughters can. As I said before, I'm not so sure my son will be able to part with his double cheese. He is a really good sport about most things, but if I gave him a veggie burger instead of his favorite takeout food, he might revolt."

Smiling, she said, "Then keep the burgers on the menu. We don't want any broken bones or broken hearts when we sit down to eat. If something is too hard to give up, then don't. Instead, give up the parts of the cow your family can live without . . . sausage and steak, for example. While you're at it, maybe you can toss out the pig and chicken, as well. Eventually, your son might be ready to give up burgers. Or not. Either way, if you stop serving the rest of the meat, you are still ahead of the game. You can also begin to substitute other options."

"Such as?"

"Well, instead of spaghetti and meat sauce, you can serve the pasta with marinara. Make bean and cheese burritos instead of beef. Vegetarian sausage tastes the same as regular sausage, and I love vegan chorizo. I've been putting it in breakfast burritos for my own family for months, and they haven't noticed the difference. Once you get going, you will be surprised how easy it is."

It was a good base for beginning my transition. Perhaps my husband and I could start first and see how it goes. Cutting meat out of our diets before changing the kids' eating habits could make it easier to work out the kinks. Teenagers can be a fickle group.

"I think I have it. Is there anything else I need to know?"

"Yes, the main reason I feel it is so important to switch to a vegetable-based diet."

"Didn't we already talk about the main reason for changing? I thought it was to help heal my body and, hopefully, prevent my family from suffering through even half of the medical problems I've had. Did I miss something?"

"Absolutely. Although that is a pretty good reason, too."

I was on a mission to heal myself from the inside out: mind, body, and soul. We were discussing the body part, so what more could there be? "Okay, I give; what am I missing?"

For the first time, she looked annoyed. "Why do you think we try so hard to compartmentalize life?" As she talked, tears filled her eyes. I felt that she wasn't just talking to me but to our society as a whole. "When are we going to realize that life isn't about one thing or another thing; it's about everything together?"

Why was she getting so upset? After all, it's just food. I felt as if I was on Mars and she was on Venus. Was she talking on a higher level than I could understand? Or was she saying something I just hadn't heard yet?

On the other hand, maybe God was trying to talk to me through Pamela. Is it possible that God talks to all of us through others? Wouldn't it be great if we took the time to listen?

I decided to stop speculating and ask the obvious. "So how is food related to all of life, then, Pamela?"

She walked over to the window by her desk and opened it. While sitting on the sill and looking out at the world passing by, she began. "Think about it, Lisa. What is food if it isn't life itself? We have become so detached from what we put in our mouths that we don't even consider its origins or its effect on us. And I'm not talking in only the biological sense."

Her passion for what she believed in was clear, even if her message to me wasn't. "What do you mean by detached? And how else is our nutrition affecting our way of life?"

"Have you ever gone on a sugar binge?"

"Sure, who hasn't at some point?"

"How did you feel after?"

"Guilty?"

"Why are you answering my question with a question?"

"Because I'm not sure what you want me to say?"

"You are doing it again."

"I know. It's kind of my thing. I've been told it can be annoying. Maybe giving wrong answers makes me uncomfortable?"

"Stop it."

"Okay, I'll give it a try. After a sugar feast, I feel satisfied and happy at first. Then a little guilty. Then I feel irritated for doing it in the first place. And sometimes sad or depressed. Eventually, I crash and just get tired."

"So sugar has biological ramifications and emotional ones, too?"

"I guess."

"When I asked you how you felt after you ate a bunch of sugar, I meant how you physically felt. You answered me with how you felt emotionally. That means you had an emotional response to what you ate, as well."

"I suppose I did. Using the term *comfort food* would be an emotional response, too, right?"

"Right."

She grew quiet and started petting her dog, who was always nearby. "Have you ever been to a slaughter house?"

The thought of it made me cringe. "No, why?"

"How about a butcher shop? Ever watched as they chop up the sides of beef?"

I remembered the meat shop of my youth. The butcher, a really fat man who usually had blood on his apron and smelled funny, was a friend of my mother. His shop always made me sick to my stomach.

"I have. It was nasty."

"Why nasty?"

"It smelled like death. They would bring in whole cow sides. You could pick which one you wanted, and the butcher would cut up the entire thing for you. It made me feel sad."

"Why do you think you had an emotional response if it is just part of life?"

"I don't know; it didn't feel right. It seemed so cruel and thoughtless."

"Not all people feel that way, which is fine. But if you do, and you eat meat anyway, you are hurting your spirit."

I laughed out loud and asked, "How can eating a burger hurt my spirit?"

She moved her chair next to mine. "Your spirit is telling you that harming animals is not something you should do; otherwise it would not bother you. If it does, then you are not living in alignment with your spiritual interests. We are all wired differently, so it is important to figure out what your personal truth is regarding your diet. If you get a funny feeling in your belly that eating something doesn't feel right, then you need to trust that. Also, ask yourself if compassion, kindness, and mercy to animals are important to you."

"Well, of course they are!"

"Don't jump to conclusions. Many people believe that animals were put on the earth for our consumption. But it isn't true for everyone. What is important is to heed your spirit and your truth; otherwise you cut yourself off from both."

Her dog curled up at her feet and sighed as if agreeing with what she was saying. She looked at him and smiled as if she knew what he was thinking. "Our mind, body, and spirit are connected. When we abuse one, the others get damaged in the process. The good news is that as we rebuild one, so the rest shall follow."

There was a sense of clarity in what she was saying. A clean body helps clear the mind, and a thoughtful and conscious mind strengthens the soul. They all work synergistically. The body is similar to a microcosm of the planet. Just as the mind, body, and soul were designed to work together as one, so were we designed to work as one with all other living things. For the first time, I was beginning to grasp the concept of the circle of life.

I grabbed a pen from my purse and wrote "Rent The Lion King" on my hand to remind me to pick it up from Red Box on the way home. Given the circle-of-life concept, it was now clear why it had always been one of my favorite Disney movies.

Isn't it amazing what you think of when the mind has no filters?

I came back to reality, trying to form a question for Pamela. "So I think I understand the body component, and Mona got me on track with the mind part. Does that mean the spirit sort of takes care of itself if the other two are in alignment?"

She looked beyond me, almost as if she might find the answer in the distance.

"I suppose it could. Or you could help it along a bit."

"How would I do that?"

"By connecting with your spirit directly. Without realizing it, we can become complacent and disconnect from our soul. Why or how that happens isn't as important as being mindful of it and reconnecting."

"Can you help me do that?"

She gave me her twinkly-eyes smile. "No. I can help you with your nutrition, but you will have to find someone else for that part."

The prospect of searching for a spiritual guide gave me pause. "That might be a tall order. How could I possibly know where to find someone authentic? I mean, for $39.95 there are all sorts of DVDs on how to be spiritual, but I seriously doubt there is much enlightenment involved in them. How would I know who is the right guide for me?"

"You are open and awake now. You will know. Just put it out there. Say a little prayer and keep your eyes open. Remember, if you build it, they will come. Right?"

Hey, that's my line.

I went home and debated where to turn next. I thought about discussing our conversation with my Coffee Club, but they didn't seem very spiritual. On the other hand, they had led me to some great people so far.

I decided to keep an open mind for the time being and see where the road might lead. It hadn't steered me wrong yet.

CHAPTER 39

The universe is full of magical things patiently waiting for our wits to grow sharper.
Eden Phillpotts

HAVE YOU EVER TRIED to control what you dream at night? There are lots of old wives' tales that say it's possible, but I don't know if I believe them. We can try drinking warm milk, watching TV, and listening to special music, but at the end of the day, I'm pretty sure that we dream what we're supposed to dream.

And yet I keep trying to do it anyway.

As I closed my eyes, my intention was to be anywhere but near an ocean. Crossing over into my sleeping world that evening, a muddled picture came into focus, and I realized I was once again walking along the shoreline, like every other night.

At least the landscape had changed. Thousands of huge crabs covered every inch of the beach. On closer inspection, I noticed tails wagging and realized the crabs had turned into puppies.

My dreams seldom make a lot of sense.

As far as the eye could see, there were kittens, as well. They were all staring at me as if waiting for me to do something.

Then it was upon us. With that all-too-familiar sound of shells turning on top of themselves, the seawater rushed back toward the horizon.

I held my breath and waited. It was only a matter of time before the tsunami reached us, ready to swallow me and all of my furry friends, erasing any trace of our existence.

Again.

Then, from behind me, I heard him. "Why aren't you running, Meliana?"

I didn't bother turning around. I knew exactly who was there.

"I'm tired of running, Melville. So tired. If that stupid wave wants to take me away, let it. I don't want to fight anymore."

Dejected, I kept my back to him and studied my feet. He gently reached around in front of me and started drawing a design in the sand with a stick. I couldn't quite make it out.

"What are you doing? Why are you here today? And why am I here again? Clearly, I do not understand whatever it is you are trying to teach me. If I did, I would probably not be having these ridiculous dreams about tidal waves over and over. This is all so futile, anyway. My health keeps slipping away like the tide. Maybe my moment on earth is supposed to be over, and I'm fighting a losing battle. Maybe I should simply let go of my tether to life."

"Oh, poor Meliana. She is feeling sorry for herself again and trying to give up."

I could hear the patronizing tone in his voice.

"Well, what else am I to do? I've done everything I could think of. I've done everything that you and everyone else has asked and followed every instruction to the letter. Nothing seems to be helping me get better. What else do you want from me?"

"Dear girl, you must observe things from a different perspective. Nothing is ever as it seems initially."

He put his hand on my shoulder and gently turned me around to face him. I was startled to see not my trusted friend, a bearded man in white, but an angelic being, hovering above the ground.

"Melville?" I was confused.

"You call me Melville, but I am called many other names by those who need me."

"Well, then, what do *you* call you?"

"I am seen as you need to see me, and I act in a way you can comprehend. I am always here for those who call on me."

"That didn't answer my question." I wanted a response I could actually understand.

"I have taken the form of Morpheus for now."

"Why? Are you really someone else in disguise?"

I figured our relationship was strong enough for my ludicrous line of questioning. After all, it was only a dream. Right?

"No, but as I said, those who ask for me will perceive the version of me they need. I take shape in whatever form is necessary. But let's return to you and your pathetic point of view, Meliana."

That was the Melville I recognized, the one who never let me get away with anything. "I forgot what we were talking about."

His glistening body floated downward. As his feet hit the sand ever so lightly, he assumed his old form.

"My point, child, is that things are never as they seem. Life is not a linear quest; it's a hologram."

I gazed at the sphere he was drawing in the sand. Somehow it was all supposed to make sense.

He had grossly overestimated me.

"How is life a hologram? What are you talking about?"

Patiently, he picked up a rock and handed it to me.

"Look at this stone; what do you see?"

"I see a stone. It has ridges on the side and a little sand in the crevices."

He flipped it over. "Now what do you see?"

I focused more intently. "There are pits in it. It looks like a little sea animal may have lived there at some point."

He leaped with excitement, and his body stayed slightly above the ground, hovering over the sand pictures.

"You got it!"

I still felt confused but joined him anyway in celebrating my vague comprehension. However, as I jumped up and down, my feet hit solid ground.

"Yay me! Now tell me what you think I got, and I will tell you if you are correct."

Surely he'd notice my trick, but I had to give it a try.

He played along. "So, what you are saying is that from one vantage point, it is just an old rock, but from another view it is . . . or was . . . someone's home. You can view an object from many different standpoints and get various understandings of it. Am I understanding you correctly, Meliana?"

It sounded good to me. "That's exactly what I was thinking. Sometimes when we stare at something for too long, we lose our perspective. You have to turn it over a few times and perceive it in another way to truly understand its complete meaning with clarity."

"Your understanding is very deep, Meliana. And perhaps that is where you need to go next."

Damn. I'd almost grasped the truth for a minute, and he had changed directions on me.

"Where do I need to go, Melville? Or do I call you Morpheus now?"

"You can call me whatever you like, because I am both of those and neither of them. As I am constant, I am ever changing, just as you are. The rock was once a boulder. At some point, it will be a grain of sand. And yet it is still the rock that we know. Life is different from each viewpoint, from all vantage points, from every angle. All we need to do is observe through different eyes, even if they are our own."

"I think I understand. When I was taking a painting class, I would be in the middle of my work, and it would appear to be a big mess. That was when I would set my brush aside and walk away for a few minutes. Upon returning, it was clear only a few changes were needed . . . a little touch here and a few strokes there and . . . voila! It was done."

"So your 'big mess' turned into a beautiful masterpiece after you viewed it with fresh eyes and decided to keep going. All it needed was a few more strokes!"

His feet came down again, and he landed in the middle of the hologram he had drawn for me in the sand.

"It is time for you to do the same, Meliana. It is time for you to view your life from a different perspective."

I gazed at the rock still in my hand. "What perspective would that be?"

He took the stone and pounded it on the sharp edge of another that lay on the ground. It split in two.

"You have done a good job of looking at the external you from various viewpoints; now look on the inside."

"Didn't I do that with Mona?"

"Yes, that is one view, but it was only scratching the surface. There are others. Your work with her reflects your responses to the outside experiences you have had in this life, but you haven't seen them from your soul's vantage point."

"How do I look from my soul?"

"You look in, not out. Search your heart in the stillness of your being. You will find the answers there."

I gazed into the distance. The sea had calmed and returned to its natural state. No tsunamis for me that night. When I turned to Melville, he was gone. The stone was gone, as well.

I started to walk along the beach and noticed the puppies and kittens had become human babies. They were still and peaceful until one started crying; it was a rhythmic sound I had heard before but couldn't place. Then another one joined the first, followed by another, until the sound was almost deafening. Covering my ears, I screamed for Morpheus to help me stop the noise. I screamed louder and louder so he could hear me over the racquet. Then I woke suddenly and realized I had been calling to him out loud as I slept.

Then I recognized the loud but familiar rhythm I'd heard in my dream. It was my husband's snoring. I got out of bed and grabbed a pillow from the chair next to me. He woke up to me hitting him over the head with it to get him to stop.

Rolling over, he squinted up at me, confusion written on his face. With his eyes at half mast, he asked, "Are you trying to kill me?"

"Not tonight, but if you don't stop eating dairy right before bed, I may tomorrow. Remember the name Morpheus for me, though. Okay?"

"No problem. Now can we go back to sleep?"

"Sure."

I wasn't sure I wanted to sleep. The problem with learning in your slumber is that you don't get a lot of actual rest. As my husband drifted off with no problem, I fumbled my way in the dark and hid in the bathroom. My dog dutifully followed. She must hate those late nights with me.

I typed in the name Morpheus on my smart phone, which was charging by the sink. It turned out that in Greek mythology Morpheus is the god of dreams; he had the ability to take any human form during the sleeper's unconscious state.

Interesting.

And a little weird that I would wake up screaming his name.

I pondered what he had said about seeing things through my soul's perspective. So many new concepts had been revealed to me since disease had taken over my life. I wondered what else in the world of healing might be out there that I never knew existed. Whenever I seemed to reach a dead end, a new modality had magically opened up to improve my life. My bet is that many options are available to us if we are willing to investigate them. I said a little prayer that my next path would soon reveal itself and kept the faith that as long as my intention and discernment were clear, I would be open to whatever followed.

After petting the dog for a minute to thank her for her company, I went back to bed. For the remainder of the night, I experienced nothing but darkness and peaceful rest. It was a nice change.

CHAPTER 40

Virtue is not left to stand alone. He who practices it will have neighbors.
Confucius

AT THE WORST POINT in my disease, I felt that I was filled with and surrounded by nothing. *Nothing* is the term that best described my state of being.

Absolutely nothing.

I was so physically tired that I spent weeks, even months, lying listlessly in bed. Any stimulus, including light and noise, greatly affected my biochemistry and ability to breathe. We had to limit the amount of time my own children could spend with me, as the smallest amount of excitement would send me into choking/breathing spasms. Most of my days were spent propped up in bed, staring at my bedroom walls and listening to the oxygen tank that pumped life into my frail, thin frame.

The slightest addition to the already agonizing fatigue I experienced daily caused my body to shut down. I would then appear lifeless, as if in a coma but conscious just the same. Often, I wasn't sure whether I was awake or asleep. Thoughts aimlessly bounced around in my head, but I was unable to grasp them. Maybe that is why my dream state became so strong. It was all I had to help me pass the time. As the days turned into months, my physical body wasted away, and my dream life became my reality.

It was very confusing, yet very clear.

Life became extremely challenging and more than a little unpredictable. I would start to feel stronger and suddenly relapse for no apparent reason. It happened again and again.

Other than my closest friends, the few visitors who stopped by had no clue how to relate to me in that state. I can imagine how difficult it must be to attempt conversation with someone who is gasping for breath, with eyes closed and a face void of all expression. Folks didn't hurry back for another visit.

It wasn't because they didn't care. They ran because they didn't know what to say or do. At least I hoped that was the case.

I felt trapped in a world of suspension. Not alive. Not dead. I was stripped to the core of my being with little to no ability to move, think, or speak.

With no other option than lying motionless, I decided to go deep within myself.

I didn't choose meditation; it chose me.

When I was a working mom with three busy kids, I knew people who meditated, but I could never figure out how they were able to fit it on their to-do list. After hearing about how wonderful they felt afterwards, I tried it briefly. Following the protocols I had researched, I attempted the Zen state they were raving about. In our very loud house, the only suitable spot was the floor of the garage behind my wedding dress. We'd married in the nineties, when big skirts were in, so there was a lot of material to get lost behind. There was no direct access from our house to the garage, so I figured it would be a while before the dog and the kids found me, typically in that order.

Following the meditation instructions direct from the Internet, I lit a candle to help me focus but soon realized that candles should not be recommended unless you use them in a well-ventilated space. We are still trying to get the smell of smoke out of my dress.

The article suggested coming up with a special word to clear the mind. I found a semi-comfortable spot to sit and began to repeat the word. It started out fine. Then grocery shopping popped into my head.

Bananas, bread, and milk.

Focus, Lisa.

Eventually, I got back on track and in the zone again. Then the dog outed me. I heard her outside the door, whining. Thoughts intruded again. *Did they walk her? I recently had the carpets cleaned, and I can't afford any more accidents. Should I call someone to take her around the block?*

My attempt to meditate had failed.

There were too many rules anyway. Meditation had to be done in a particular type of space and on a daily schedule for a predetermined amount of time. And there was that special word to repeat during the process.

What was up with that?

Why couldn't I tell anyone the word I used? Would something bad happen to me if I did? Was it like those chain letters we get as kids that tell us to make a bunch of copies and pass them out quietly, or our life will turn to ruin?

Needless to say, in the days before illness claimed me, all meditation meant to me was more on my to-do list, which was already exploding at the seams.

Now in the clutches of disease, I decided to try again on my own terms. My illness erased the ongoing chatter that once consumed my head; it calmed my mind, allowing me the space to see into my soul.

Looking back, I now understand that the meditation rules are there to get you started. But they are merely guidelines; if anyone says differently, find a new teacher, book, instructional video, or whatever is telling you what to do. We are all in different places in our lives, and there are many streets that can lead us to our destiny. I decided that my job was not to sit passively in the passenger seat of my own car but to start driving.

I simply needed to find a road map to help me reach my destination.

And the key to start the car.

CHAPTER 41

Every moment and every event of every man's life on earth plants
something in his soul.
Thomas Merton

THE FEW FRIENDS who were brave enough to find ways to spend
time with me had incredible patience. But between my slurred,
inaudible words and inability to move much of the day, the best we
could do was lie in bed together and watch TV. Minnie and I had
spent the morning watching a program about a guy who'd found
enlightened guidance through an acupuncturist. Rather than the
typical acupuncturist who deals with physical ailments, that one
could place needles in certain spots on the body and open doors to
all sorts of spiritual experiences for the pokee (the acupuncturist is,
of course, the poker).

Minnie, who is incapable of relaxing, was hemming a pair of
jeans and surfing the web to come up with curriculum ideas for her
homeschooled children while she watched with me.

Enthralled with the concept of needles producing mind-altering
experiences, I tried to say, "Wouldn't that be awesome?"

"What?" She looked up blankly as she finished a French cuff on
the pants. There is nothing mini about her energy. Just watching her
was exhausting.

I tried again to get the words out, but they emerged more slowly
than before.

"Wouldn't—it—be—great—if there—were—such—a thing—as an
ac—u—puncturist— who could—expand—your mind—and open—you
up—to all the—answers—the universe—holds?"

Just getting the sentence out was grueling.

"There are. They're called esoteric acupuncturists," she remarked as she continued her multitasking and ignored my obvious speech difficulties. "They are trained to open blocked channels in your energetic body and help you connect to your spirit. It raises your vibrational frequency to a higher level and can move you along the path of enlightenment."

"How on earth—do you know—that? You—grew up—in Scranton."

"Yeah, but my grandfather on my dad's side was raised in Japan. Very old school. He loved to talk about esoteric stuff. He was big with the needles, too. It used to freak me out a little. But who has time to think of weird concepts like that anyway? I barely have time to think about what I'm going to make for dinner. I've decided to do the Meatless Mondays thing for the family. I've been researching it. You know, going vegan one day a week is going to help save the planet."

"If anyone can—save the planet,—it will be you,—Minnie. Is your—grandfather —still—around?"

I had plenty of time to think about weird concepts. All the time in the world.

"No; he's dead. But my Uncle Mikio practices esoteric acupuncture not too far from here."

I tried to sit up straighter but collapsed under the weight of my head. "Do you—think—he would—see me?"

"Sure, but why? Your problem is physical, not spiritual."

"Maybe. But what if—it is more than that? What if—all our physical issues—have some spiritual—and emotional—connections, — as well? Wouldn't it be better—to look at—the issue—from all angles?"

"If that were the case, then why can you cure cancer with chemotherapy alone? Wouldn't a disease just stick around if you had to clear it from other levels, as well?"

"I don't know. Maybe that is why—sick people—tend to get sick again. Maybe it is—because they have—something they haven't looked at—on another level,—so their bodies keep circling around—to disease. Or maybe—they start to look at life—differently—because of chemo— and clear up—the other levels—that way. I don't know—too many cancer patients—who haven't—been changed—by the process."

There were a lot of maybes in our conversation. Maybe it was because we were on to something. Or maybe it was just me questioning everything I thought I knew. I sensed that there were things going on at different levels in my psyche. There are all sorts of reasons why stuff happens to people. This particular concept was worth investigating to see if that was true.

I'm pretty sure Minnie heard what was going on in my head. "Look, we will never know why things happen, but if you want to see an esoteric acupuncturist, I will make the call to my uncle. You have to promise to just go with the flow with him, though. He is a little different from me."

I was mildly concerned. "Different how?"

"You will see. I don't want to give you any preconceived ideas. I will drive you there and back if you want. The rest is up to you."

The rest was up to me. I could live with that. Even though I was no longer in the driver's seat, I was still able to navigate my life from the passenger side. I suppose we can never really control our circumstances, but we can control how we respond to them once we find our internal compass.

CHAPTER 42

For what you call destruction is only transformation,
the aim for which is the renewing and amelioration of living beings.
Allen Kardec

ONE WORD CAME TO MIND when I first met Mikio: conundrum. He fit the definition perfectly. Mikio did, indeed, present confusing and difficult questions. It was impossible to estimate his age, he spoke in riddles, and his Japanese accent remained very strong despite the fact that he'd spent much of his life in Los Angeles. He also possessed a collection of very sharp needles. Needles have always made me extremely nervous.

As soon as the word *conundrum* crossed my mind, I longed for a glass of wine. Not so coincidentally, Conundrum is the name of my favorite white. I was certain a few sips would calm the growing apprehension I felt.

My new acupuncture therapist worked out of offices located behind his house, which was in a neighborhood that became ground zero during the 1992 South Central riots in LA. Seeing the bars on the windows of many homes in the area, I thought it might be a great idea to install them at my own house when the kids became teenagers; they might decrease the likelihood of anyone trying to sneak out at night. I was pretty sure the bars on those particular windows were meant for something entirely different, however.

Minnie and I arrived for my appointment in her family-sized SUV, which screamed "White suburban Mom on board." Mikio was standing at the door, waiting for us. He wore white linen pants and a white tunic. His hair and long beard were also white. Leaning on a bamboo cane, he seemed lost in time, a man who would look exactly the same in any given century. As he summoned me inside, I glimpsed the tattoo on his arm. It appeared to be a Harley Davidson. How did I keep finding people who live in opposites? Didn't they know there are rules about how we are supposed to be in this world? I was pretty sure that if you were living in one of the more dangerous areas of the city and sporting large tattoos, you weren't supposed to be an ancient, wise Asian acupuncturist.

But I could be wrong.

He greeted me with a warm smile and gave me a hug that took my breath away. Literally. For a small, fragile-looking man, he was amazingly strong.

"Greetings, my fellow traveler! So happy you journey finally find its way to me. I have been waiting for you."

He gave Minnie a hug, too, and graciously sent her on her way.

As she backed down the driveway, she yelled out the window, "I'll pick you up after I finish my carpool. You are in good hands. Have fun!"

I waved goodbye and turned to Mikio, contemplating his statement about waiting for me. Did he mean that in the metaphorical sense, or had I lost track of the time and arrived late for our appointment?

"You have a very nice home and office. Have you lived here long?" I asked casually as I tried to figure out how a little Japanese man ended up living between two of the roughest housing projects in the country. It really was a beautiful house. The Japanese gardens in the courtyard were as peaceful as could be.

"Yes. Live here many years since land call me to it. Mother Earth shows what we need and where is needed."

I wasn't quite sure what he meant by that. Maybe Mother Earth was the name of his real estate agent.

"Come in. Sit down." As he assessed me, he appeared to be looking through me and around me rather than at me. "I see you very hot on outside of body, but you insides is rice cold; you very freezing."

His accent was hard to make out at first, but I found it endearing after I got the hang of it.

"You rie down so I can take better look at you."

I did as he said and lay on the table, covered with a sheet. He was gazing at a point just above my head.

I began to worry that visiting him hadn't been such a great idea after all. Who was he and what did he see that I couldn't? I decided to relax for the time being and roll with it. When in Rome, I suppose. "Whatcha looking at?"

"Many blockage, many broken parts, very disconnected. Spirit has left building. I see big black mess around heart and kidney, too."

My confusion and skepticism became stronger, but I was willing to give him a little latitude since he was related to a trusted friend who wasn't going to pick me up for hours. "And that means . . ."

"When Supreme Controller is sick, there is no one to guide, to love, to lead. No one to give orders or set boundaries. No warmth or happiness. Life no fun. With no leader on throne, every official cry out in distress. That when fear and panic take over. All this happen without you knowing. This when we get sick."

That sounded interesting. And if I managed to fully comprehend what he said, I might find some truth in it. Maybe I should stop my inner chatter of doubt and start the session again with an open mind.

"So you are saying I am at war with myself? And who is this Supreme Controller, anyway?"

"You heart. The love we receive from fire element, from you heart, bathe every part of life. It warm our spirit and give us communion with God. You so cold inside, no fire. Old cold, from many lifetimes. When we connect to fire, we feel love of self and others. We need reconnect you to source of Supreme Controller. The divine within connect to the divine without . . . one in same."

"And how are we going to do this?" Although I still wasn't completely clear what *this* was, or if I was ready to buy into that stuff, I was willing to keep my overabundant judgment at bay until all the facts were in.

"We do it by acupuncture and meditation. We get you back to you spirit. Solid spirit; it just not attached. We hook you up to vitality again. You strong girl, no problem."

After we were done talking and he had left the room, I lay on the table thinking. Before I got sick, I would never have entertained the idea of seeing someone like Mikio. Heck, I didn't even know people like him existed. And if I had run across one of them, I would have written him off as peddling some New Age thing . . . even though there is nothing new about acupuncture or meditation.

Is writing something off without fully investigating, just because we don't understand it, really to our benefit?

Our Western mentality would probably judge Mikio's concept of healing as nonsense or a big waste of time, because it isn't steeped in medicine, tests, or drugs. Were more of those modalities, which weren't really working, the best solution for me?

And did any of what he said go against the religious principles I was raised to believe?

The answer that came to mind to those questions was "I don't think so." At least not in that moment. Listening with discernment means we listen with both our head and our heart to find the truth. Although Mikio spoke words I didn't fully understand, they didn't ring untrue, which felt like a green light to at least explore this new idea.

People have been healed with therapeutic methods other than Western medicine for thousands of years. What kind of egomaniacs have we become to discount or discard something just because it doesn't fit our way of thinking?

I decided to push through my own prejudice and explore the Eastern way of healing and trust Mikio to show me a new path. I had read somewhere that we all have an inner voice that speaks to us if something doesn't feel right. As long as we listen closely to it and follow our minds and hearts, we will be safe.

Faith is a beautiful thing. I had asked for a guide to help me learn how to look at myself from deep within, and I'd found one. I wasn't sure how I ended up in the care of a man with such intrinsic knowledge, but he filled me with hope that I was on the right road again.

CHAPTER 43

Believing is seeing.

Anonymous

AS I CONTEMPLATED the meditation process Mikio had shown me, self-doubt clouded my mind again. Meditation is great for people who want to find inner peace and become more self-aware, but I had serious medical problems that were developing rapidly. My weight had dropped to numbers I hadn't seen since middle school, when I was four inches shorter, and I was becoming weaker by the day. Was a spiritual search the best thing to be trying at that point? I was starting to seriously question how it could help me heal.

Instead of following the many rules he'd given me for searching my soul in the comfort of my own home, I opted to stall a bit longer and paint my nails. They had been looking pretty shoddy, and I loved the new color my daughter had bought. It was called "I'm Not Really a Waitress" red. I thought waitressing sounded better than quietly waiting for a transformative miracle that might or might not occur.

After delaying the inevitable for as long as possible, I put away my manicure kit and, with nothing else to do, got back to business.

Mikio and every other guide who'd helped me along the way said I had all the answers I sought within me. Was I flunking my life's test because I hadn't been able to access those all-powerful, elusive solutions?

Patience is such a frustrating notion.

Determined to give the "finding my life lesson in this disease" concept one last try, I changed things up a bit and moved my practice sessions to another location. As Mikio had suggested, I found a place where I wouldn't be interrupted and could focus.

I took a chance and meditated in my bathtub. If it didn't work out, at least I would be relaxed and clean. I'm pretty sure if I weren't human, I'd want to be a fish. There is something about floating in water that makes me very happy.

My daughter loaned me a tape with music that's supposed to put the brain into a theta mode, which she told me is a meditation state. She had used it when she was drawing and enjoyed where it took her artistically. With the lights dimmed and the music playing, I hesitantly lowered myself into the tub, attempted to clear my mind, and waited for the magic to happen. And waited some more.

Either the people on the Internet who rave about the life-changing aspects of meditation are full of bull or I was not grasping the big picture. I wasn't seeing any picture at all, for that matter.

I thought about the saying "If at first you don't succeed, try, try again" but opted to ignore it and finish washing my hair. My mother used to tell me it was better to step away from a situation to gain some perspective than to beat your head against the wall attempting to figure it out. Accepting her advice, I decided to wait until my appointment the following week when I could ask Mikio what I was missing.

When Minnie and I arrived for my next session, I staggered into his office and plopped onto his treatment table. I had to carefully lift my wobbly legs to get them aboard, as they weren't cooperating.

Struggling to breathe lowered my voice to barely a whisper. "I'm doing everything you told me to do, but nothing is happening. What am I missing? Do you believe God is trying to tell me to move on to something else?"

Mikio waved his hand in front of his face like he was batting flies away. "No. No. Don't be silly. You think too much. That you problem. Want results. Americans! Always thinking, never understanding. Instant gratification or throw in towel."

I tried to roll to one side to see him, but the motion made it even harder to breathe. "What do you mean?"

"My point is you not need a point. Relax and let go of expectations. Stop thinking, start being. You so full of thought, you lost in own head. Too much judgment going on in there. Relax. Stop all the worry about what you and others should do and think. Just *be* for little bit and will come clear. I put needles in you. You get the point."

I might not get the point, but I did get the irony in his last comment.

Lying motionless on the table, I did my best not to think. I didn't think about the things I could no longer do or the cost of my healthcare or what my doctors or Christian friends would say about me having esoteric acupuncture. I didn't think about the family I'd let down by my months of bed rest. Most of all, I didn't think about the numerous needles in my head, predominately on my forehead, which Mikio called the third eye.

While listening to the music that played in the background, I heard the beating of my heart, the rhythm of my breath, and the . . . *sound of whispering in my ear?*

At first I thought I was imagining the faint sound of the voice that called to me from a distance. Ugh . . . I was thinking again.

Pushing those ideas out of my mind, I focused on breathing and tried to deepen my inner hearing. I silently mouthed a question. "Hello? Anybody there?"

Yep, that sounded as psychotic as I'd thought it would.

"I'm here, Lisa. Go deeper, and you will find me."

Hmm. Male voice. Powerful but gentle. Faint. Almost like a dream but strong just the same. Okay. I'll bite.

Taking a deep breath, I dropped into hyper focus, releasing all control and melting into the table. My body totally relaxed. It was a familiar feeling, the kind I often experienced right before I fell asleep, as if I were falling. I let it all go and stayed totally in the moment.

After a few minutes of nothingness, I started drifting through what appeared to be a tunnel. Was it possible the nothingness I had been feeling all along was a gateway to another dimension in my mind that I didn't know existed? Maybe I hadn't given that space an opportunity to develop.

Oops. Well, no time like the present.

I saw a spiral, spinning with a kaleidoscope of colors that got stronger and brighter as I looked closer. Taking another breath, I released all expectations and walked through the spectrum, totally immersing myself in the colors as if they were flowing through and around me simultaneously.

Then I saw him. At least, it seemed that someone was there. Looking with my mind's eye, I sensed a form in front of me, an oddly familiar presence. He was an ancient soul with a kind face, completely dressed in white. It was as if I could see him without actually seeing him. I felt his warmth as strongly as his presence. It seemed very safe and peaceful there, wherever there was.

Was I dreaming? Probably not, because I still heard the background music and the street noise, but they seemed far away in another dimension. Was that what I was supposed to feel in a meditative state?

So far, so good, I guess.

"Hello?" I said again, not knowing what else to say.

"Hello, Lisa. I told you that you would find me."

"You did? Have we met before?"

"Do you remember that night in the hospital when you were deciding whether or not you should wake up? That was me talking to you. I've been talking to you in your sleep for most of your life. You haven't been able to hear me while awake until now. Without realizing it, you lowered the volume on my voice years ago."

"Oh, sorry. Maybe we could start over. I vaguely remember the hospital experience, but I could use a little help on the volume concept. Where are we exactly?"

"We are here."

"Where is here?" I desperately wanted a better perspective of where I was and what I was doing there.

"In your mind and soul. I am somewhere between here and there, between this world and the other. You reached me through your spirit. Your internal compass knows the way to me, but you have to be willing to seek me."

"Internal compass? Like my conscience?"

"Partly. Everyone has a higher self that connects to the One if they choose. I am the conduit to the highest of powers. If you remember how to listen, you can regain the knowledge lost during life's experiences. Your job, if you wish to accept it, is to retrain your ears so you can listen to your internal world while awake as easily as you listen to the external world."

"How do I do that?" I imagined I was seriously getting on that guy's nerves.

"All in due time, Meliana."

I was a little hesitant to correct him about my name for fear he might realize he was talking to the wrong person and move on. Still, I felt compelled to set the record straight.

"My name isn't Meliana." Although for some reason the name did sound vaguely familiar.

It is here."

"Why?"

"Because your spirit is named Meliana."

"Why?" I felt like a two-year-old asking redundant questions.

"That is your purest name. It is how we refer to you."

"Why? Wait . . . we?"

"Yes, but that is for another visit. For now, you need to find the road in. Into your mind, into your body, and into your soul. Build a highway and then connect all three with strength, for it is your path to wellness."

"How do I build this road with strength when I am so weak?"

"Jesus said, 'If you bring forth that which is within you, what you bring forth will save you. If you do not bring forth that which is within you, what you do not bring forth will destroy you.'"

"Did he tell you that directly?"

I was simply trying to grasp some idea as to the guy's hometown.

"It's in the book of Thomas. Look it up."

He was not providing much help in the perspective area. I had many, many more questions to ask, but I sensed Mikio calling me back to reality. I felt myself being pulled through the kaleidoscope of colors. Suddenly, I sensed the weight of my body, heard the music from the stereo, and smelled the oil that had been rubbed on my forehead. I opened my eyes to a grinning Mikio as he leaned over my face to remove the rest of the needles.

"Welcome back! You have good trip?"

I sat up as if I'd been shocked.

"What was that?" I shouted.

He looked puzzled. "What?"

"What . . . or who . . . was that? I don't know for sure what just happened, but it's possible I am going crazy."

"Why you say you crazy?"

I lay down on the table again. "Wouldn't I have to be crazy to talk to people who aren't there?"

He laughed. "Maybe some are, but pretty sure you not in that category."

"Why not? I was having a conversation with a man who clearly wasn't here. Sounds a little crazy, right?"

He shook his head. "No. Not right. Did you actually hear him with your ears?"

"Hmm. Not really."

"If you hear something and didn't hear with your ears, then you hear with your heart. That better anyways. Truer."

"Truer? Truer than what? Logic?"

He paused to choose his next words. I was pretty sure he was searching for terms to dumb down whatever he needed to convey. "We have two sides of brain. Both understand but in different ways. Western culture teach one way, the logical, left-brain way. They believe is better than the other, because it can come from books or Internet or school. Something tangible. That not always the case. Other cultures have seen much learning from right side of brain, too, where intuition lives. Americans forgot how to listen different way."

"Is that what I experienced? Did I learn to listen through the other side of my brain?"

"Sort of, yes. You listen through you heart. That little voice is intuition. We can ignore or fear it because some church say is evil but is only a sense of knowing coming out. I told you. You already have all answers you need. All peoples do. Need to remember them and not judge process. Is difference between learning and understanding."

I doubted that I'd learned or understood any of that conversation, but it seemed profound for some reason. It was one of those things that makes sense on a gut level. I enjoyed that type of learning. It was much easier than all the reading I did in college. I was eager to talk to that guy again. Being reassured that I wasn't crazy or possessed opened the floodgates to a host of questions to ask the being who called me Meliana.

Tucking my arms against my body and closing my eyes, I reestablished myself on the table and asked, "Can you return those needles to their previous positions, please? I have some unfinished business."

I felt I'd been pulled out of a beautiful dream by an offensive alarm clock telling me it was time to face the world. That world sucked. I wanted to experience the new world and go there again. Wherever there was.

"No can do, boss. You done. You saw what you supposed to see. Now have to do own work."

"What work do I have to do on my own? You are the one with the needles. I just have to lie on this table with an open mind. I can't do it by myself. I'm not even sure I can keep my mind open all by myself."

He laughed. "Maybe that first thing to work on. Change brain waves, too, and you will find paths back in. You can do, you smart cookie."

I so wished he would stop saying that.

"I have to change my brainwaves, too? Is that even possible?"

"Of course it possible. You already doing it. You figure it out. I see you next week. You strong girl. It what saves you. By the way, I really dig your toes polish. Very nice color."

As I left Mikio's office, a wave of peace washed over me like a soft, warm blanket. I wasn't sure where we were going with the process, but the goose bumps on my arms and the sense of deep contentment were enough for me to realize there is more to life than the naked eye can see. Truth is truth. Once we are awake, we not only see it but feel it, too.

CHAPTER 44

Find a place where there's joy,
and the joy will burn out the pain
Joseph Campbell

FOLLOW-UP APPOINTMENTS with Mikio were temporarily put on hold. It had been a terrible couple of weeks for me physically, and I'd been admitted to the hospital again. I was hoping Mikio could offer me some relief through acupuncture now that I was finally home and more mobile. He greeted me with a warm smile but was more somber than usual. His look of concern was unmistakable as he stared into my chest, which was about eye level for him.

"Oh, gosh, you in bad shape. What happen?"

"I've been having trouble breathing lately. It's part of this dumb disease. Apparently, my diaphragm decided to go on vacation but didn't find anyone to fill in for it. It's kind of hard to take in air when the muscles in your chest area aren't working."

"What take you breath away?"

"Myasthenia Gravis, the autoimmune disease I have took it away. It happens sometimes."

"No, what element?"

"What element? What are you talking about? In our last session, we discussed knowing versus learning and listening versus hearing. As complicated as those concepts are, I thought about them the entire time I was in the hospital, and now you throw this element stuff into the mix? Man, you are hard to keep up with."

Trying to breathe and talk at the same time made me extremely dizzy. The lack of oxygen to my brain was taking its toll.

"Not really. It all work together. Like I say, what element?"

I didn't have a lot of patience for learning something new at that point. My objective for our appointment was to simply stop feeling so terrible. "Um, I dunno. Can't you just help make this crappy weakness go away? I'm so tired. To-the-bone tired."

Realizing he was talking to someone who was clueless about Eastern concepts and in no mood for a philosophical conversation, he tried an analogy. Pulling a wooden match from his pocket, he lit it and said, "Watch. Wood transform into charcoal as long as flame goes down the match. Look closer now; underneath, you see tiny bit of water. It evaporate and transform into hydrogen and oxygen. See, I give you example of main elements of life as we know it: Earth, which is wood here, fire, water, and air. All need to work together to make universe and everything in it operate in harmony like match does. Each element flow with the other. You not flowing. You stuck. Too full of one part, not enough of other makes you out of balance. You not breathing. Not enough air element. Means you overcompensating with another. Which one throw you off?"

I tried to calm myself enough to understand the idea and see where or if it fit in my world. I wasn't sure which element was taking over, so I thought about how it felt not being able to take in a full breath.

"Well, it feels like there is something heavy sitting on my chest all the time."

He jumped up and down. "Then that it! Earth taking up too much space. Need more room for air. If over-abundant fire, there would be burning in lungs; with water, you would be wet coughing. You have to consider why earth took over for air. Fix it, and you feel better. Easy."

Easy? Maybe when you think like an ancient Chinese medicine man but not so much for a softball mom.

I looked at my chest, trying to find some sign of the earth element paralyzing it. I saw nothing unusual. "And how do I do that?"

"You figure it out. You strong. I put needles in now. Help you remember."

My kids hate it when they ask me a question and I respond by saying, "You're smart; I'm sure you can figure it out all by yourself."

I was starting to understand just how annoying that could be. And why did Mikio keep talking about remembering? To remember, you need to have experienced something already. Or could he be talking about a deeper, inner knowledge again? He clearly had more faith in my ability to understand intrinsic concepts than I had in myself.

Luckily, I did feel physically better when we were done and was able to take in a full breath after my treatment. However, nothing mind-blowing had happened during our session, and I was sort of sad that the beautiful man in white hadn't come to visit me in my mind. There were many questions I'd planned to ask him if he decided to stop by. Instead, I spent my time on the table in a deeply relaxed state, despite the dozens of needles in my body.

Unfortunately, relaxing didn't help me understand why there was too much earth and not enough air in my being, nor did it show me how to balance the elements. Maybe that would come in time.

During the drive home with Minnie, I sensed a shift in my perception and looked at the people around me with different eyes. Did the needles have more of an effect than I'd realized? I was trying to see how and why we become out of whack with each other and ourselves.

It got me thinking. Are we born in perfect balance in the first place? Or is it our primary goal in life to find middle ground as we walk through our individual stories? Is life like a video game that has us jumping over one thing and ducking another to stay alive while gathering points for every successful attempt? Or do we come out of the gate a bit off and try to learn how to be in the world while working on whatever issue we cosmically chose to fix?

Does any of that even make sense? I turned off my brain for a minute and looked at the hands of the dear friend who was driving me home. Minnie is always so busy, and her life is starting to wear on her physically. Does that mean that she has an excess of the fire element and needs to offset it by learning more about peace, which would be in the water element? Is that part of her cosmic quest?

Are we all born with a life plan designed to bring our existence into equilibrium? Is this what *God's divine plan* really means? As many times as I have heard about the concept in church, I never really understood its potential meaning until then. Was I given the gift of illness to learn something about peace in the middle of chaos? Is that my divine plan? And had I just considered my illness a gift?

The ideas that ran through my brain amazed me. When I was healthy and my goals were more basic, like trying to remember to pick up the dry cleaning on the way home, I would never have considered such lofty concepts. Could expanding my mind be one of the reasons I had arrived at that particular junction in life? Was I supposed to think deeper, to gain more wisdom in areas I never knew existed?

Who knows?

All I knew for sure was that overthinking had again added a headache to my list of current physical issues. Before going to bed, I included Advil in my nightly bucket of medicine and decided to ponder these new ideas in the morning.

Mornings always seemed to bring more clarity, especially when my friend joined me in my dream state during the night.

CHAPTER 45

Never let fear decide your fate.
Awolnation

THE NEXT DAY, I SPENT some time with a cup of tea and the sheet Mikio had given me that described each of the elements. Reading the paper over and over, I looked for some clue as to why I was so out of balance and how to fix the problem. The information seemed pretty straightforward. I just wasn't sure what to do with it.

WATER: Solitude, privacy, introspection, philosophy, mystery, truth, honesty, anxiety, nervousness, insecurity

Positive Characteristics: Compassionate, loving, forgiving, sensitive, easygoing, modest, flowing, deep, truthful, creative, wise

Negative Characteristics: Overly sensitive, weepy, dependent, indifferent, lazy, insecure

FIRE: Self-expression, emotional extremes, empathy, extroversion, attention-seeking, sociable, talkative

Positive Characteristics: Energetic, enthusiastic, courageous, daring, faithful, quick, funny, flirty, lively, cheerful

Negative Characteristics: Stubborn, greedy, jealous, angry, resentful, flighty, nervous

EARTH: Caring, supportive, nourishing, family-oriented, stable, grounding, "mother hen," worrier

Positive Characteristics: Reliable, punctual, stable, persevering, wise

Negative Characteristics: Greedy, sensualist, materialistic, stodgy, narrow-minded, irritable, tough, aggressive

AIR: Objective, intellectual, communicative, mental agility, dreamers
Positive Characteristics: Joyful, humorous, communicative, intelligent, intuitive, diligent
Negative Characteristics: Gossipy, boastful, spendthrift, untruthful, selfish, fickle

Mikio viewed imbalances in the body as elements that, once identified, could be adjusted. It seemed easier said than done. Mona had used the realms to seek disparities. The language was different, but the goals were the same: to find where we are out of kilter and bring us back to the center of our being. That much I got.

What was it Mikio had said about me . . . that I was too full of the Earth element and lacking in Air? How did that apply to my life?

I attempted to break it down. If having the Earth element meant being caring, supportive, nourishing, family-oriented, and a worrier, then an overabundance of Earth would lead an individual to worry excessively and be overly supportive and invasive in the lives of others. Mona would describe that type of person as codependent, someone who has no boundaries and always puts the needs of others first, even at her own expense.

I could see some truth in that for me.

Mothers are inclined to do that anyway, but we aren't helping anyone if we get lost in the process. We end up miserable without knowing why. A strong woman never thinks that will happen to her, but it kind of sneaks up over the years, especially if she isn't working outside the home.

What about the air part? If the Air element means being objective, intellectual, and communicative, then not having enough probably means that somewhere along the line, I lost my power and my voice.

Having a family full of strong personalities has its blessings and its challenges. There is a biblical passage that says "iron sharpens iron," but sometimes it is too exhausting to keep up and be sharp all the time. It is often easier to simply retreat to the drawer where the dull knives live.

It was starting to make sense.

If my spirit is naturally strong and vocal, and I am not exercising it by speaking my truth, my voice becomes weak. That may create an inability to breathe, both literally and esoterically, which is a huge part of my disease. If I am over caring or worry excessively, I feel the weight of the world on my shoulders, which makes me feel weak and powerless . . . the other part of my physical disease.

I took a break from the heavy contemplating to get something for the ongoing pounding in my brain. So much wisdom and deep thinking were starting to make my headache worse. Of course, it could have been the post-IV migraine I typically get. The timing was about right.

As I tried to ignore the throbbing in my head, I better understood how an emotional or mental stimulus could produce a physical response. I understood how it could work in reverse, as well. My autoimmune disease attacks not only the physical body but seeps into the emotional and spiritual body. It's as if the disease had to show itself in a physical realm so I could see the harm I was doing to myself on an emotional and spiritual level.

I knew the mind, body, and spirit are connected somehow, but to actually see what each is doing and how it affects the other was powerful. We tend to compartmentalize the many actions or thoughts we have in a day, but each and every thing we take in or do affects us by either building up or breaking down our bodies. When the hair on my arms rose, I knew the concept was ringing true for me.

Although I didn't believe that my actions were the leading cause of the disease, enough evidence existed to see their contributions. More importantly, I knew I could use that information to accept my past actions and learn from them instead of judging myself for them. It was a fresh start, with new insight as to how I want to live my life in the future.

Hopefully, working with Mikio would help me open up on all planes, lifting some of the weight from my chest, allowing more of the precious life-giving air into my lungs, and helping me achieve better balance.

I thought about how, not that long ago, I would have dismissed the entire concept as some weird voodoo idea without giving it a second glance. Looking through the notes from my dream journals, I reread an entry about the various interpretations for a shell. On one hand, it can be a piece of art decorating one's house. For a sea creature, the shell itself serves as a home. I contemplated how much my own home had changed. Internally, I felt like an entirely different person. My compassion for others and for myself had grown exponentially, as had my understanding of the bigger picture. Externally, our home life had also changed dramatically since I started this journey. Commando Mom had given way to a softer, hopefully more understanding mother. The kindness that had blossomed in my family's hearts made my own soul melt with pride.

Without opening our minds to different ways of perceiving, we can easily dismiss concepts that can help our understanding of the world around us, as well as ourselves. I had begun to realize that we are the ones who control the limits of our own growth.

How many times do we learn about an innovative idea and discount it because it's foreign to our way of thinking? Some even take it further and consider any idea that is beyond their frame of understanding as dark and sinister. I believe our job is to approach new concepts with discernment and figure out which ones ring true for us without immediately judging them. Truth really does set you free if you have faith in it. Fear of the unfamiliar will only keep us locked in a little box with others who share our narrow thinking.

I had developed a willingness to be open to everything, while understanding that some ideas would not be right for me or my health. My mother always said there was nothing wrong with looking; we never have to buy. I had developed the ability to view my world with a little distance, too, like a scientist who tries to figure out what combination produces the best results.

If no two people are the same, how could we possibly believe there is only one method of healing that works for everyone?

In retrospect, I suppose that statement could apply to almost anything in life.

CHAPTER 46

*At any given moment we have two options: to step forward into growth or
back into safety.*
Abraham Maslow

I ARRIVED EARLY for my weekly chat time with the girls and
watched the crowd place their orders. A customer stood in line
across from me as he waited for his double espresso. He appeared
ready to explode with anger as the poor barista fumbled with the
order, spilling it as soon as she finally finished. I thought about what
Mikio had said. The man was probably not in total balance, or he
would have been a bit more compassionate about the situation. His
face was red with fury as he stormed out of the coffee house, yelling
about the idiots that worked there. Mikio would probably say he had
too much fire in him and needed more water to cool down and let
life flow.

I decided to play a game with myself to see if I could figure out
which element was the most predominant in each of my friends.
Making up head games was something I'd learned to do while
spending all that time in bed staring at the wall. Sometimes those
games carried over into the real world.

Posing a question to Minnie first, since she was right next to me,
I began. "Minnie, what would you like to drink?"

"Oh, can you get me a latte? No, wait, I think I'll have a
cappuccino. Never mind. I was reading about the health benefits of
green tea the other day . . . lots of antioxidants in it. I guess I'll go
with that."

If my interpretations were accurate, Minnie most resembled the water element, because she flowed with the tides and never stuck to one thing for too long. She also formed many of her opinions from an outside source.

I tried it again. "How about you, Cheryl?"

She answered without looking up from her Blackberry. "Black. I'll just have black coffee."

Cheryl always knew exactly what she wanted. She was also inflexible. If I were to pick an element closest to Cheryl, it would be earth. As Mikio said, when earth is not in balance, we see people who are unable to change or who are stagnant in their energy.

I continued. "Maude, what would you like to drink?"

"I'll have . . . did I tell you what happened to me the other day? I found out at the last minute that I was going to be in charge of the decorations for the kids' school prom. Are you kidding me? How am I supposed to organize that? Do you know how many things I have to do? Oh, that reminds me, I need to make an appointment for a mani-pedi. Anyone want to join me?"

Maude may be most aligned with the air element and be slightly lacking in earth to ground her.

Once our drink orders were filled, we sat at our usual table. As I looked at the beautiful faces before me, I thought about how we are on such diverse paths yet still good friends. It made me wonder how often our lives are touched by those from different walks.

Listening to the usual chatter, I smiled inwardly and said a little prayer of gratitude for these dear women and for everyone else who had shaped my existence. Who would have thought these random people, put together by fate, would have a hand in defining who I was and what I might become?

My friends were my fellow travelers, and I appreciated them more every day. Perhaps we are all fellow travelers walking in step along different paths, never knowing what is around the corner. I used to think life is a race to the finish. I finally understand that the process of getting there truly is the most important part.

Dr. Habib said that we are perfect in our imperfections. That must mean that our imperfections define who we are. God gave us these traits to help us grow into the people we are to become, so those imperfections must be perfect. Before I got sick, I would never have given that statement a second thought, but now that I've had the time to slow down, the concept has changed the way I relate to myself and everything around me. I am no longer filled with disappointment because I can't do all that I used to. Neither am I the over-controlling person who tried to force everyone to see things her way. It is through our flaws that we can see our character and show society that different isn't bad or shameful; it is merely different.

There are many things I have had to let go of because they are too hard for me to do physically. On the other hand, my new life is just as rich with other experiences and ideas that would never have happened had I stayed well. Trajectories are funny things. With a subtle change in course, we can shoot for the moon and end up on Mars. Mars may not be where we were headed, but it could potentially be even better than our original destination if we are open to what is in store for us there.

CHAPTER 47

Nothing endures but change.
Heraclitus

AS OUR SESSIONS progressed, Mikio's energy seemed to change. It was more mindful and deeper in some way. Of course, it could have been my energy transforming instead. I wasn't sure. I just had a sense that something felt more soulful . . . if there is such a thing.

During one meeting, I watched him while lying on the table, ready for my next treatment. His focus was even more intense than normal. I often thought it would be interesting to crawl into his mind and hang out for a while. It would probably be the only way I could comprehend how he thinks.

"Is everything all right, Mikio?"

He looked at me thoughtfully. "I really like you new shoes. Very funky."

I chuckled to myself. Who would ever have guessed he was thinking about my shoes? Or that he paid any attention to fashion? On second thought, hanging out in his head might be too much for me and my little brain.

"Thanks. Anything else?"

"Yes, you all okay. Better than okay. The light is flowing through veins and filling body back up with vitality."

I laughed again. "Is that why I've been gaining so much weight? It's almost back to normal. And my strength is coming along, as well. I finally said goodbye to my cane the other day. It made me very happy."

His tone was not as jovial as mine. "The body underweight before because it have to die and recreate itself on cellular level for you to live. Now the sun shine in your cells like springtime after long, hard winter. You open now. Blossoming."

His imagery made me smile. "I've been very receptive to this process. I've even enjoyed the shifts I have experienced from those needles all over my body. Who would have thought that could happen? I was the ultimate baby when it came to shots as a kid."

"No, that not what I mean. You chakras open. I see violet ball on top of head. It so beautiful. Also, there is halo of white around it. Very nice."

Closing my eyes, I took a moment to check in with myself. He was right; even though I couldn't see the colors he saw around me, there was a freer feeling that hadn't been there before. I felt it from the core of my being and knew it wasn't just my mind that was less restricted but my soul, as well.

Then my brain kicked in again.

"Glad to hear that, but what do I do with this new feeling?"

"What do you do? Nothing. It not a *do*, it a *be*. It means you open to life. Open to spirit. You ... open."

"I get it. I'm open. Now what?"

"Why you always have to see *what*? Concentrate on *why*. That when you see purpose in life. Why you here. You try and see more, think less, be very present."

See more, think less, be very present. I wondered what Mona would say if she could translate Mikio's language into her own. She would probably think it meant I was more accessible to myself and my surroundings, with less judgment. I wasn't thinking about all the other distractions but enjoying every moment instead. However, I was still having trouble with the life's purpose part of his comment.

"I get what you are saying, but I'm still not sure I totally understand my purpose yet. How will I know when I've found it?"

"Just know. You been coming here long enough to understand. I think you know, too. Just not accept yet."

"Or maybe I simply haven't seen it?"

"You see. It right under you nose all the time. You want help understanding?"

"Yes, I want help understanding."

Lord knows, I wanted help understanding.

"Okey dokey. You go see Mandaza. He help you. It time for fresh guide anyway."

"And who is Mandaza?"

Maybe I should have asked *what* a Mandaza is. I never knew with Mikio.

"He my friend. African shaman. Very powerful. Very beautiful. You see. You like."

Shamanism now? What next? Dead chickens being waved over my head?

Wait. There I was judging and discounting an idea before I knew anything about it . . . again. Mind chatter can be a dangerous thing. If you don't catch what you are thinking and bring it to the surface, it can get away from you quickly.

Did seeing a shaman sound a little out there for me? Definitely.

A little scary? Maybe. Probably more intimidating than anything. African shamans aren't typically in the wheelhouse of people to whom I would normally defer. But, then, neither were esoteric acupuncturists, and that seemed to turn out rather well.

Did I trust Mikio and my own discernment?

Absolutely, to the first part. Regarding the second part, I would say I was in the beginning phases of trusting my own intuition. I agreed to do a little research of my own. If what I learned rang true for me, then I would call the African shaman.

It was time to practice what I was preaching to myself in my own head. Fear of new and different things had run my life up to that point. So far, it hadn't gotten me where I needed to go.

Does fear ever move us forward? It is a great ally when we are in real danger and something to pay attention to in the discernment process, but do we really want it ruling our existence?

I found fear exhausting and decided to try something different. Replacing fear with faith in myself and my dear friend Mikio, I opted to try another new path and at least be open to thinking outside the box. Why not? It was getting increasingly claustrophobic sitting inside those four walls anyway.

CHAPTER 48

The soul always knows what to do to heal itself.
The challenge is to silence the mind.
Caroline Myss

SCHEDULING MY FIRST appointment with Mandaza was like planning a visit with someone from another planet. I had no idea what to expect or if it was even possible to effectively communicate with him why I was there or what I was looking for.

From my research, it was clear he wasn't from my part of the world.

My homework had started with the basics. Since I didn't know what a shaman was, I checked the dictionary and found that shamans are spiritual leaders who have special powers, such as prophecy or the ability to heal.

That was interesting but didn't really explain much, so I looked him up on the Internet. I was surprised to find that he had his own website. He even had a YouTube channel.

Who would have thought?

I learned that Mandaza is a Nganga, a Bantu shaman or medicine man from Africa. He travels through North America for much of the year talking with groups of people to give them a greater understanding of the interrelatedness of healing, peacemaking, and community.

Mikio had described Mandaza as a warm and generous teacher and a healer with magnificent gifts. He also said he was a man of deep and profound love, laughter, and wisdom.

Who could resist a chance to speak with someone who possesses those qualifications?

When we met in person, I saw a gentle giant who was as powerful in stature as he was soft in spirit. His dreadlocked hair was black as coal, with naturally frosted white tips.

He wore dress pant cut-offs and a tee shirt with "Visit British Colombia, Canada" printed across the front.

Mandaza towered above my head as he engulfed me in his arms. With a powerful, deep voice, he said, "My dear friend, I am so happy to see you today. I love you very much and want to do whatever I can to be of service." His glistening white teeth shone brightly against his jet black skin when he smiled at me. He was truly beautiful, in every sense of the word.

After inviting me to sit, he asked, "How are you, dear girl?"

My response was immediate and almost robotic. "I'm great, thanks."

He paused a minute as his face softened. "Then why do I see tears behind your eyes?"

Suddenly, there was a knot in my throat. The tears he saw from deep within surfaced faster than I would have cared for. My emotional filters seemed to disappear with every kind word that came my way.

I felt raw and completely vulnerable in that moment and had nothing left to give but brutal honesty. Although I had just met Mandaza, I opened up to him more completely than I had to anyone before, including myself.

"I'm not sure why I'm still alive. Everyone else who was struggling with their own health issues alongside me has died. It would be so easy to let go of my hold on life, but then I look at my family and can't bear leaving them, so I fight for another breath and another day. I don't know how much longer I can keep this up, though. It gets harder and harder, both mentally and physically."

I looked out the window to the trees in the garden as I pondered my life. "Once I saw a little sapling caught in a violent storm. The wind blew so hard that the poor thing was bent completely over to the point of breaking, leaves tearing from her branches. Most of the time, I feel just like that tree."

Closing my eyes, I slumped deeper against the wall, which was keeping me quasi-upright as I sat on my floor pillow. "I'm tired of being tired and stripped down to nothing but bare branches."

He reached toward me and put his massive hand over mine. "Fair enough, my dear. Now tell me why you are here with me, child."

It was a great question. Why was I there? Because I was so desperate I would try just about anything? Because I was weary from being teased by feeling almost human again for a few days and then having the rug pulled out from beneath me when I became too weak to move? Because Mikio said it would be good for me? Maybe it was a little of all of those. But, more importantly, I think I was there because something deep within called me to be there. Somehow I knew that larger-than-life man who felt oddly familiar could look into my heart and awaken the process of initiation that would remove the obstacles between my soul and the heavens.

Wait. What? Where did that thought come from?

My own mind had begun to speak an unfamiliar language without providing me with a dictionary.

I decided to drag myself out of my head and give him the obvious answer to get things started, but what came out of my mouth startled me.

"Well, I've been sick for a while now. According to my abysmal blood tests, I should be in the hospital, barely breathing, if at all. But I seem to have tapped into something that defies basic chemistry and keeps me going. For reasons I can't explain, I'm still here, and it feels as if I will ultimately be the one who heals myself in some capacity. I just don't understand how yet."

He drew a deep breath, taking in my comment, and closed his eyes. "Go on."

The words came to me as if someone had put them there for me to hear. "It seems that most of the light switches in my head are on now, but there are still a few dark spots. I am looking for a way to flip them on. The medicine I take from my Western doctors is helping, but it isn't my cure."

I was fascinated by the information spilling from my heart. My soul had taken over the conversation, and I was merely listening to the sound of my voice.

Mandaza's eyes flew open, and a huge grin spread across his face.

"Correct! What you speak is the truth. The doctors' medicine is not going to cure you. This disease you have is the message of a different calling. We all have a purpose in life. Many search for it. Some run from it. Most don't even know there is such a thing. Your guides want you to discover that purpose. They have been sending you many messages you haven't understood for a very long time."

After finishing his sentence, he appeared exhausted.

Trying not to overstate the obvious, I asked, "If it is clear that I am not understanding the message, wouldn't it be better to put it in a simpler, more understandable form?"

His eyes were void of any expression. Whatever vision he saw had nothing to do with our surroundings. He appeared to be in a trance when he started speaking.

"You see, child, the water spirits I carry flow between two worlds, this one and the world of our guides. You came here so that I can help you decipher the code of your messages."

"I did?"

"Silence now, child. It is time for me to talk to your spirit guides. They will help me bring into focus what has been blurry for you."

So far he was on point. Life does get a little blurry when you have no idea what you are looking for . . . or at.

The room became uncomfortably silent. I was never very good with long, awkward pauses, but I was scared to move a muscle for fear he would not hear the answer I was seeking. When he finally spoke again, his voice sounded distant.

"I see you have been getting a dream for a very long time now."

Startled, I felt as if a bolt of electricity had just run through my body.

"Yes! I have been dreaming the same dream almost every night for over eight years. That's amazing! How did you know that?" It felt like my soul had opened up to him, and he could read it clearly.

"Quiet, child, I am with your spirits now. These dreams have changed recently. You haven't been having them as often, have you?"

My voice was barely audible. "No."

"I will explain it to you this way. Let's say Mandaza loves you very much. He misses you and is thinking about you constantly. He wishes to speak with you, but he is on the other side of the world and cannot call you, so he sends you an email. You read the email but do not respond. He still wants to contact you, so he sends you another email. You read this one, as well, but you do not respond. What does Mandaza do?"

"Stop sending emails?" I felt a sense of dread, like I'd blown it.

"Correct."

"But I didn't understand the emails. I've been trying to figure out the dreams for years, but I still don't comprehend their meaning."

"Then you need to ask the spirits for another dream, a simpler one that you can understand."

"Oh." *Why didn't I think of that?*

"Tell me this dream now, child, and I will help you decipher it."

I shut my eyes to clearly see my story.

"It's the same every time. I am walking on the beach, and there are children or young animals playing in the sand everywhere. I look up and see a giant tsunami coming in, and I try to help them reach a safe spot as the water begins its assault. Once the wave comes, I desperately hold onto a tree or something sturdy as the sea sucks me to its depth. I struggle to keep my grip, but the power of the wave pulls me under. I usually wake up just before I drown."

Mandaza erupted in a howling laugh. "Of course. It makes perfect sense."

"Really? Enlighten me." I had my doubts that any of it made sense but was willing to give it a try.

"The water spirits form one of the most powerful forces in the spirit world. They have been trying to send you a sign for many years. When you didn't respond, they called you back to them for more instruction. You are resisting by not letting go. This struggle is partially responsible for the spiritual side of your health issues. The dreams didn't work, so they had to up their game to get your attention."

"They have my full attention now. What is it they want?"

"Your maternal energy is very strong. In your dream, you protected the children on the beach before you worried about your own safety. The guides are showing you your calling in this life. You are here to heal the world's children."

I started to laugh.

"Oh, is that all?"

Me? Who are we kidding? I can't even get my own children to listen to me.

"It seems daunting, but it is not. The children of the world desperately need healing. Where I come from, children are used as human shields during battle. Children are also used for slave labor and sex trading in many countries. They have no voice and are defenseless; they need healing. This is your calling. When you answer this, you will be better."

"That's ridiculous. How would I even begin to do something as huge as that? I barely have enough energy for my own family, not to mention myself."

"I don't know. That is up to you and your spirits to decide. Before you go to sleep tonight, ask your guides for forgiveness. Tell them you are sorry you have not heeded their call, but you did not understand what it was they wanted of you. Then ask them for another dream, one that you can understand. Ask them how it is that they want you to be this person. Tell them you will listen intently; you just need clarification. Do you understand this, child?"

"Yes. But I feel a little like that guy in the Bible who stood behind the wine barrel and hid when God asked him to fight an army in His name. I am sure you must be mistaken. I don't think any spirits would intend for me to do something that grandiose. I'm just not someone who could handle helping the children of the world."

"You will understand in due time. Just have faith that all will play out as it is intended, but you must release all of your control."

I hate it when people say to release all control. I relish control. I will admit, however, that it hasn't worked for me so far.

Mandaza then walked around behind me and said, "Now let me feel your pain." He started rubbing my back with his massive hands.

I made a mental note to get a massage soon. It had been a while, and his soothing touch felt pretty good.

"Oh, so many needles in your body. I can feel them. They are in me, as well, now."

"Sorry." I didn't want him feeling bad, too.

"No. This way I know where to go. You have many needles in your nerve endings. And your kidneys are tired. They have been working very hard, haven't they?"

"I take a lot of medicine. They should be pretty tired."

"I will help calm your body. Release your pain into my hands. My body is heating up. This means the water spirits that live inside you are very thirsty. You need to replenish them. You haven't been drinking enough water, have you?"

Wow. That was totally correct, too.

"No, I haven't. It is hard for me to swallow, so I don't drink much."

I suddenly felt ashamed for not properly nourishing my own body.

"They ask that you drink. Flush out your system. Help your kidneys do their work, and feed the spirit that lives in you."

That part I could handle. "Okay. Anything else?"

"Go to the beach today. Play with the children there. Connect with them and your own inner child. Your spirits will give you the information you need at that time and also tonight as you sleep. Do not worry. It will all come to you in due time. I love you and only want the best for you, my dear."

He finished our time together by saying a prayer over me and then retreated into the other room.

It had to be more than coincidence that he had recommended playing on the beach. It was the last day of school for my youngest daughter. I already planned to drive her to a beach party after school.

On my way home, I thought about what Mandaza had said. We all have our own purposes in life, our own truths. Life's little puzzle was figuring out what that truth is and following it with conviction. It seemed so simple yet so impossible. Shouldn't there be a *Finding Your Purpose for Dummies* book out there somewhere? Things would be much simpler if we got some type of personal owner's manual when we were born. That way we could be clear about which path to take and when to take it.

I couldn't wait to pick up my kids and their friends and hang out on the beach with them that afternoon. We all needed a little fresh air and play time.

Fresh air always cleared my head of chatter.

On the other hand, maybe I should have been listening more closely to all that chatter.

CHAPTER 49

Feeling my way through the darkness
Guided by a beating heart.
Avicii

THE KIDS AND I stayed at the beach until the sun reached the horizon that afternoon. The view was spectacular and the smell of the ocean hypnotic. After piling into the car, tired and sandy, we all went home longing for showers and sleep. Once the house had been shut down for the night, I lay in my own bed saying a silent prayer to the designer of my dreams. I asked for forgiveness for not understanding the meaning of the message for so long. Clearly, I was not in this spiritual school's gifted program. Taking Mandaza's advice, I asked for a dream that would allow me to clearly see my purpose in life and how to fulfill it. I also asked for help in releasing the ropes I had clung to for so many years and the fear that accompanied them. If the tsunami wanted to take me home, I would go willingly and learn whatever it wanted to teach. My body melted into the mattress as I closed my eyes and crossed over to my other world.

Softly, the beautiful music infiltrated my very being. It was everywhere and nowhere. The melody surrounded me with an unrecognizable but gentle tune. I walked along the corridor of an enormous stone building. In the distance was a large neon sign. Peering through an opening, I saw what looked like a train or subway station. It appeared very old and dilapidated but beautiful just the same. The music bounced from wall to wall, the sound resonating from every orifice.

People were everywhere, mindlessly running to their destinations and listening to the sweet sound. As I entered the next room, I heard a harsher tune, that of babies crying. They were hungry, so I tried to feed them, but their bottles held thick milkshakes instead of baby formula. It was undrinkable through the nipple. Running from the room, I searched for someone to help me, but the robotic crowd offered only blank stares and continued shuffling by.

Then I saw him.

"Melville?"

He wore a symphony conductor's tuxedo and waved a baton wildly over his head, prompting imaginary musicians to play a tune.

"What are you doing, Melville?"

His eyes remained closed as he filled the air with sweet sounds from his musical commands. "Do you hear the music, Meliana? Isn't it beautiful?"

"It is. I don't recognize it, though. It sounds a bit like Bach but not exactly."

"Exactly! Not exactly. Do you know why? It's because it isn't exactly Bach. Did you know that if you change or extend a single note in a piece of music, it changes the sound of the entire opus?"

"I guess I never thought about it, but I understand how that could happen. Where are you going with this?"

"Even the minutest shifts can cataclysmically change the flow of things. If we are mindful of what we are doing and make small changes in our way of being, the result will be exponential. It's simple math."

I began to comprehend his message. "So you are saying that I don't have to be overwhelmed by a goal. I only have to take tiny steps toward it, and the goal will take care of itself?"

"Exactly. The important things are the intention and mindfulness of the process. If it is your truth and you believe with all your heart in what you are doing, you can be fearless as you walk along your path."

I closed my eyes and listened to his imaginary symphony. The melody of the initial song rested faintly on the new version. I felt the rhythm as he adapted the original to create something new. Ever so subtly, he turned it into his own personal truth. Then the music faded, and so did Melville.

His beautiful song filled my mind as I returned to the room with the crying babies. I felt helpless and lost as to what to do for them. They were hungry but turned away and cried harder every time I offered them their bottles. I sat next to one and started eating an apple. As I cut off a small piece, an idea formed. I handed the bit of apple to a child to see what would happen. He popped it into his mouth and ate it gleefully. Then he ate another and another. The poor thing had been starving. Until then, I hadn't thought out of the box as to how to feed them. I cut more apples and handed out pieces to the other children. They couldn't eat them fast enough.

Then I heard Melville's familiar voice whisper in my ear once again. "Meliana, you have to nourish the babies. They need pure, clean food, not substances that clog and frustrate them. They have been fed lies their entire lives. Their drink has been made from an obsolete formula developed long ago that doesn't work for the children of today. It was created by selfish men whose concern was more for their own profit than the welfare of those they served. The children are hungry for what they really need: the truth."

I woke suddenly as if someone had thrown cold water in my face. Sitting up in bed, I thought about my dream, wishing I could return to it. *Baby steps for babies.* Was that the key to my goal? Was I the baby or the caregiver? By changing a simple thing like removing the chemicals from the babies' diet and replacing them with fresh, pure food, their bodies were able to get the nutrients they needed. Maybe it was symbolic for all of life. When we are fed lies, our bodies and minds become bloated and corrupted. We end up becoming the lie. Truth is clean and pure. Could that be what Mandaza meant when he said I had to save the children? Am I to simply show them what their truth looks like?

There were many questions for which I had no answers, but at least I had some food for thought. *Food for thought.* I chuckled to myself at my newfound wisdom, even if it arrived as a silly metaphor.

I turned to my husband in bed and said, "Small changes provide cataclysmic results!" Although my guide had used those words before, it felt as if a light bulb had turned on in my head when they fell out of my mouth. In that moment, I truly understood the meaning from the depths of my soul.

He half agreed as he rolled over and drifted back into his coma. Instead of hiding in the bathroom, I stayed in bed and pulled out a notebook and pen to record my lesson. My husband was sound asleep, so I didn't think he would mind. Suddenly the task Mandaza bestowed on me didn't seem so daunting. We all have a purpose in life. When we find it, it may seem overwhelming. But if we make small, mindful changes with intent and belief, we can get closer, and, possibly, achieve exponential results.

I was sure that Mandaza's intention for my life wasn't to heal all the children of the world, but I could start by healing my own inner child and work from there. I was much more comfortable biting off smaller, tangible pieces of my goal. I figured by staying open, maybe I could help others, as well, as I started to heal. The concept seemed simple enough, and breaking it down made it much easier to wrap my head around.

Mandaza's mission for me had seemed a little ridiculous at first, but the more I thought about it on a smaller level, the truer it rang. The best way to change anything is to start with ourselves. I could certainly begin to heal my own little girl. As she heals, so do those around me. As others heal, so do those around them ... and on and on. It only takes one match to set an entire forest on fire. He could be on to something after all, if we start with baby steps.

CHAPTER 50

Strength does not come from physical capacity. It comes from an
indomitable will.

Gandhi

NIGHT AFTER NIGHT, I paid close attention to the details of my slumber. Before I went to bed each evening, I would lie in total stillness, no TV or music to disturb my thoughts. I set my intention to fall asleep in peace and hopefully understand the lessons that appeared. My goal was to listen to the voice deep within, which so desperately needed to be heard. There was a sense of urgency for me to understand what Mandaza had said about my dream life. By not fully comprehending the messages, I had already wasted so much time.

At first I heard nothing but the beating of my heart and the sound of my breath. Doubt crept in as I contemplated what I was doing in the darkness of night. I consciously pushed away all thoughts to concentrate on relaxing fully. It wasn't until then that I was able to fall asleep.

Suddenly, I felt myself falling. The landscape seemed vaguely familiar, like I was experiencing déjà-vu. Down the rabbit hole I tumbled, just as Alice in Wonderland once had, until landing on solid ground.

But where was I?

Although I sensed nothing around me but blackness, I experienced no fear. I stood still, waiting. Mysteriously, a torchlight appeared at my feet, and I picked it up. It began to burn brighter as I started to walk, surveying the terrain around me. Then I saw them staring at me curiously. Frozen and confused, all that fell from my lips was "Hello?"

I really seemed to be Alice at that point.

Without a word, they motioned for me to look around. A beautiful waterfall emptied into a crystal clear pond nearby. As the light became even stronger, I saw lilies floating on the water and birds flying overhead. Wandering around, I found a large oak tree and sat down; the grass was cool and comfortable.

I turned to see that hundreds of wild animals had followed me. They graciously greeted me in their habitat as they surrounded the tree. It felt warm and welcoming, as if I had been invited to some fabulous party.

I sensed his presence before seeing him. "Melville?" It had to be my dear friend.

Emerging from behind the tigers, he called to me. "I'm here, Meliana."

He sat beside me as I asked, "Where are we?"

"You tell me. This is your creation, remember? We manifest our own classrooms in this world. Where do you think we are?"

"I don't really know. Maybe we are deep beneath the earth's surface in a safe place. I like it here. It's comfy and cozy. Feels like home."

I was making it up as I went along, but it somehow rang true.

"And the animals?"

After hesitating for a minute, I responded. "I think the animals are here to guide me. Maybe they are some of my teachers."

He jumped to his feet and did a little dance in the grass. "Works for me. What are they doing?"

I stood up and turned in a full circle, examining the terrain as the magnificent creatures moved to different areas in the savannah. "On one side of the stream, they are standing near some people who appear to be scared. Folks are running into the water and climbing trees to get away. On the other side of the stream, the same animals are standing near a different group. Those people are petting and playing with them. They are in total harmony."

"What is the difference between the two groups?"

I knew the answer somehow. "When you trust your inner voice and follow truth, the rest sort of takes care of itself. Your senses become more in tune with life, and there is no need to fear new situations. The second group checked out the circumstances and realized they were in no danger, while the first group panicked because it was an unfamiliar situation for them."

He walked into a stream, splashing wildly like a small child, and asked, "What does that statement mean to you?"

"It means that if you listen to your gut and have faith in your instincts, you won't be suspicious of others or worry about their intentions. You will know how to handle yourself intuitively and can act accordingly. Some scenarios look innocent but can be very dangerous, and others look worse than they really are. When our focus is dialed toward truth, we will know the difference and how to handle any circumstance."

"Exactly. Those who don't listen to or trust their little voice are filled with doubt and worry. They become paralyzed with fear when trying to make decisions, because they don't want to make a bad or wrong choice. Eventually, they become suspicious of the world around them and shut down. On the other hand, individuals who have faith in themselves are more open and confident. They can look at everyone and all situations with discernment, because their internal compass is connected to the heart and brain. They don't simply see a situation; they experience it, as well, and the truth is clearer."

"So if we fully believe in ourselves, we can experience limitless thinking and be open to fresh ideas and situations?"

He floated out of the stream, completely dry. "And . . ."

"And . . . if we don't have confidence in our own discernment, we eventually think everyone is out to get us and close ourselves off to life. Our world gets very small then."

"Yep. That's how we become paranoid and angry. The more confidence you have in that small voice, the more open and confident you become. And the more confident you are, the more you trust it. You're able to perceive the truth in everything. The deceivers of your world come to realize this, as well, and won't be attracted to you anymore. They will intuitively sense your personal strength and know that you see right through them."

As we talked, a few of the animals surrounded us again. There were only elephants that time. They smiled at me with their eyes, as if telling me something important. They seemed to be in agreement with our conversation. I was in total alignment with that wonderful place and hoped to visit again soon.

The colors faded as the dream slowly slipped away. I was sad to see it end and tried to hold on.

Melville whispered gently in my ear one last time. "Let it go, Meliana."

As soon as I woke, the details of the dream became fuzzy, but I remembered feeling safe and nurtured. I grabbed my journal and wrote without thinking:

Have faith in yourself and the voice you hear from your gut. Those with a lack of inner trust and confidence will somehow look fractured, not solid. They will manipulate and lie, because their internal compass no longer points toward truth. We can sense when others are not strong and whole if we listen with our heart. Self-trust comes from discernment, which is your inner dialogue connected to your soul.

The next morning, I read what I'd written while half asleep. I looked up elephants in my dream dictionary after sensing their importance. I learned that they have long been revered as wise and benevolent beasts. In Hinduism, the elephant-headed deity, Ganesh, is honored as the destroyer of obstacles. He is said to clear away difficulties and bring life to fresh endeavors.

Maybe they were trying to tell me something, after all.

It didn't make complete sense, because I couldn't remember all of it. I did, however, get the gist of my lesson. Listening to my soul and releasing the fear of what others might think of my viewpoint have always been issues for me. They say developing self-trust is like working a muscle. The more you do it, the stronger it becomes. I certainly hope that is the case.

I thought about all that I'd been learning from my many teachers. Everywhere I turned, I discovered a novel way of looking at something, a different perspective. It seemed as if I'd been traveling the road less traveled for some time, yet everything was fresh and innovative. As weary as learning sometimes made me, the lessons I picked up along the way were priceless gifts I could carry into eternity.

CHAPTER 51

SOMETIMES I FEEL as if I am continually slipping down a long, steep waterslide. The experience can be thrilling, scary, painful, and exciting simultaneously. If I open my eyes on the way down, I see the world flash before me in slow motion, with complete clarity. This helps me understand that the vantage point from which I am viewing my surroundings is unique to that particular tick in time. My task is to simply observe, enjoying each moment and staying as present as I possibly can.

Maybe we should all take it slow and stay in the moment.

Metaphorically speaking, we slosh down the waterslide of life collectively. Since there is no prize for reaching the end first, why rush? I'm pretty sure no one is any further ahead anyway. We are merely tumbling side by side, viewing the same situation from our many different perspectives.

What's important is to stop in the midst of a moment and view our fellow travelers with encouragement rather than judgment. Each smile we give shows them that we carry the faith that any obstacle can turn into wisdom if we allow it.

Forrest Gump's mama was correct when she said, "Life is like a box of chocolates. You never know what you're gonna get."

Life is all about choices, too. We may not have the option to choose what we find in our box, but we do get to decide how we are going to eat our chocolates. The way we behave in challenging times is up to us. We can empower ourselves to become students of our lives or fall prey to the events we encounter.

Our journeys can be very dark, and often we feel lost and alone. Fortunately, they can also be filled with great beauty and peace. We simply need to look beyond the suffering and float above our situation to find harmony in our story. My diseases forced me to consciously choose how I wanted to respond to life. There are times when we are forced to make tough decisions we would prefer to avoid. Heaven knows, I could have taken the easy route and let myself slip away. Instead, I decided to persevere and learn from my circumstances so that I could grow into the person God intended me to be.

Winston Churchill once said, "Never, never, NEVER give in." If I were brave enough to get a tattoo, that saying would be inked across my forehead. Well, maybe not on my head but definitely somewhere obvious to remind me daily to forge on. I've discovered that there will always be a light at the end of the tunnel as long as I don't give up the search.

If you are breathing, you will eventually deal with some type of predicament you would rather not face. You may become sick, have financial issues, be hurt physically or emotionally, or even lose the ones you love. We encounter rivers that carry us where we least expect. We must remember that although we don't control the current, we do govern our own rudder. No matter how overwhelming our situation may seem, there will always be a moment of clarity as we sail through the dark waters, a moment in which we can find our north star for direction.

Mikio was right. With perseverance and faith, my spirit had miraculously blossomed. I was finally open to love, to living fearlessly, and to finding my inner strength. For so many months, I prayed for a *normal* life, but what I ended up with was something extraordinary. I asked for the moon and was given the universe instead.

For that, I am forever grateful.

EPILOGUE

Consider it pure joy, my brothers and sisters, whenever you face trials of many kinds, because you know that the testing of your faith produces perseverance. Let perseverance finish its work so that you may be mature and complete, not lacking anything.

James 2-4

WHEN I STARTED WRITING this book, I believed that by the time I finished it, I would be completely cured. Somehow, I thought that putting ideas about my experience on paper would heal my body so I could get on with living.

Crazy, right?

Well here's the really crazy part. It kind of did. It just didn't happen as I pictured it.

But, then, does anything ever turn out exactly the way we thought it would?

As I sit by the ocean today and gaze at the reflection of the sun on glassy water while birds fly overhead, I truly do feel healed. I may not be able to run alongside the joggers who pass by me, but I am strong enough to embrace all that the world has to offer instead of mourning what I can no longer do. Before disease, life was more about striving to achieve what I didn't have. The glass was never full enough. This journey has shown me that everything I need has always been right in front of me. I just never took the time to notice. When I was running half marathons, I envied the runners who completed full marathons. There was always a nicer house or car, better cookies made for the school bake sale, or someone who earned more than I did at work. And on and on it went.

What an exhausting existence. I saw firsthand how accurate the term *dis*-ease really was when it hit me. The lack of *ease* with my life took a little time to show up on a physical level, but when it did, I had the opportunity to wear the frailty, which I'd always felt inside, like a flashing neon sign on the outside for all the world to see. How appropriate that myasthenia gravis literally translates from Greek to "grave weakness." I don't think there could have been an autoimmune disease more appropriate for me than that one.

Now that I have slowed my pace, I can celebrate and be grateful for even the smallest things that happen throughout the day. I have also been able to forgive my body for "failing" me, appreciating its nuances. I can now look with love and acceptance at others, too, instead of jealousy.

Healing comes in many forms. It can occur in the tangible, physical sense, which is wonderful, but that may be the low hanging fruit on the healing spectrum. True cures cover all aspects of our being: mind, body, and soul. It's the sense of peace we feel deep within us, knowing that whatever form our life takes in any given moment, we are exactly where we need to be.

Even if that place isn't where we thought we wanted to be.

I don't believe for a minute that bad things happen to us as some divine or karmic punishment. I think our trials are provided so we can learn and see how resilient we are while still being compassionate to ourselves and others. What I have gleaned through all this medical nonsense is to truly live every day as if it were my last, because that just might be the case.

I wonder what would happen if we all lived like that?

It's possible we would love more and fight less. Forgiveness might be more common than retribution, and greed would be replaced with generosity.

My house rings with laughter more often than it ever did before I got sick, and I thank God that He showed me how to open my eyes to a wiser way to live. I no longer judge myself or others, because I understand that we are all trying to figure it out . . . whatever "it" is. Life is simple now, in all its complexities.

We are our best teachers when we choose to be students of our lives. I challenge you to take a good look at what is going on in your world and find the truth and the lessons in it. You don't have to wait for a critical illness to force you to stop and reflect.

Eventually, everyone's body will deteriorate. No one lives forever. But our souls are eternal, and mine is more grounded in truth, love, and the divine energy that can heal us all no matter how broken we feel.

The great Paul McCartney once recommended that we "take these broken wings and learn to fly."

I am finally learning to do just that.

Namaste.

PAY IT FORWARD

Isn't it time we took our lives back from disease? With every purchase of this book, I will donate a copy to someone struggling with chronic illness or their caregiver. Simply go to WellnessWarriorOnline.com/WarriorBook to learn how you can gift this book to a friend or loved one. Alone we are strong but together we are invincible. Help others become warriors too. Join the tribe so we can all heal together.

ABOUT THE AUTHOR

Lisa Douthit is an Integrative Health Consultant who is passionate about healing from all perspectives. After struggling with multiple bouts of cancer and autoimmune disease, no one understands the physical, spiritual, and emotional rollercoaster better than she does. Somewhere between contracting lymphoma and her Myasthenia Gravis diagnosis, she made it her mission to understand the lessons available to us through illness. Also, as a homeopath, Reiki Master, Theta practitioner and through expensive nutrition education, she learned how to recreate herself and others from the inside out.

Lisa currently lives in Southern California with her husband and three children. When not working or handling her own health, she loves spending time with them in the Eastern Sierras discovering uncharted roads in the summer and skiing in the winter.

She also enjoys finding new vegan, gluten-free recipes to make for her family and friends. She is very involved with her favorite local nonprofit organization in Long Beach, CA, C.O.A. (http://www.coalongbeach.org, donations welcome), which provides over 100,000 free meals annually to homeless and very low income families. She and her daughters can be seen serving breakfast to the guests on a weekly basis.

You can touch base with Lisa at the following sites:

wellnesswarrioronline.com

twitter.com/lisadouthitww

lisa@wellnesswarrioronline.com

facebook.com/wellnesswarrioronline

pinterest.com/lisadouthitww

MORE GREAT READS FROM BOOKTROPE

Burnt Edges by **Dana Leipold** (Contemporary Women's Fiction) A story based on true events that proves strength can emerge in the most horrific of circumstances.

Tea and Madness by **C. Streetlights** (Memoirs and Poetry) C. Streetlight's memoir, Tea and Madness, is a collection of prose and poetry separated into the seasons of her life. As her seasons change, she continues trying to find the balance of existing between normalcy and madness.

A Stunning Accusation by **Sarahbeth Caplin** (Contemporary Women) In Sarahbeth Caplin's New Adult novel, A Stunning Accusation, Adelaide Scott is about to discover that the truth – in all its forms – is complicated, and not at all what she expects.

The House on Sunset by **Lindsay Fischer** (Memoir) A collection of reminiscences, scattering the ashes of two broken homes and putting them to rest. Each chapter offers a different glimpse inside the cycle of intimate partner violence, where honeymoon phases and traumas coexist.

Discover more books and learn about our
new approach to publishing at **booktrope.com**.